2023 ✓

No Time to Panic

Also by Matt Gutman

The Boys in the Cave

NO TIME
TO PANIC

How I Curbed My Anxiety
and Conquered a Lifetime
of Panic Attacks

MATT GUTMAN

DOUBLEDAY
New York

Book design by Maria Carella
Jacket image by erhui1979 / Getty Images
Jacket design by Michael J. Windsor

Library of Congress Cataloging-in-Publication Data
Names: Gutman, Matt, 1977– author.
Title: No time to panic : how I curbed my anxiety and conquered
    a lifetime of panic attacks / Matt Gutman.
Description: First edition. | New York : Doubleday, [2023].
Identifiers: LCCN 2023000750 (print) | LCCN 2023000751 (ebook) |
    ISBN 9780385549059 (hardcover) | ISBN 9780385549066 (ebook)
Subjects: LCSH: Gutman, Matt, 1977– —Mental health. |
    Panic disorders—Patients—California—Biography. | Panic disorders—
    Popular works. | Panic attacks—Popular works.
Classification: LCC RC535 .G88 2023 (print) | LCC RC535 (ebook) |
    DDC 616.85/2230092 [B]—dc23
LC record available at https://lccn.loc.gov/2023000750
LC ebook record available at https://lccn.loc.gov/2023000751

MANUFACTURED IN THE UNITED STATES OF AMERICA

1 3 5 7 9 10 8 6 4 2

First Edition

To Daphna, Libby, and Ben

Contents

No Time to Panic

Prologue

The healer told me to pull up my pants leg, baring the inside of my ankle. Her name was Brandy. On the floor of her closet-sized office, she offered a short invocation for our journey, then lit a stick of incense, blowing until it glowed red. Carefully, she pressed the incense into my skin, sizzling a row of four equally spaced blisters. The blisters rose like tiny biscuits. With a penknife, she then scraped off the tops of the blisters and placed tiny patties of frog poison into these so-called "gateways," to cook into my exposed epidermis. The patties comprised the toxic secretions of the giant monkey frog, which indigenous peoples in South America call *kambo* and have been using as a cure-all for dozens of generations.

You may have heard of a toad you smoke, whose venom, when dried and inhaled, rockets you through the cosmos aboard a velvet spaceship. Kambo is derived from a different amphibian, whose secretions keep you closer to earth—your face rarely travels more than a few inches from your puke bucket. The violent purges it induces are believed to heal everything from addiction to Alzheimer's. It's popular enough these days to keep multiple kambo studios in Los Angeles in steady business, including this one in Beverly Hills.

With my "gateways" open and the frog slime seeping into my system, Brandy and I waited. At this point, the discomfort felt tolerable, like the second day of a stomach bug. But moments later, she flipped the little frog patties to flush fresh poison into my system. Almost instantly, shock waves of nausea hit me. My skull felt like it was being inflated with a bicycle pump, my heart raced, sweat sprang from my pores, and the walls of Brandy's shoebox office crept closer.

Kambo typically takes you from feeling fine to fluey in seconds, and pumps enough fluid into your face to mimic botched plastic surgery. (The initiated call it "frog face.") As I rocked back and forth with a blanket over my head, praying my body would finally begin purging this poison inside me, disappointment crept in: I had hoped to feel sicker.

That's because kambo had re-created a suite of symptoms I had actually experienced on hundreds of previous occasions. *I know this feeling,* I said to myself. *This is what a panic attack feels like.* And maybe because it didn't hit me with the full barrage of panic symptoms—which also includes tunnel vision, foggy brain, shortness of breath, the inability to swallow, and an impending sense of death—kambo didn't seem so bad.

To get me to purge the three quarts of water she had had me drink before the ceremony, and to kick-start the healing that kambo advertised, Brandy pulled out a V-shaped blowgun. She packed one end of the blowgun with a pulverized South American tobacco called *mapacho,* then carefully inserted the business end in one of my nostrils. She put her mouth on the other end and blew, shotgunning the wad of snuff into my sinuses. It's the nicotine equivalent of smoking a pack of cigarettes in the space of a few seconds, while inhaling smelling salts for good measure. She packed the blowgun again, drew a breath, and shot another wad into the other nostril. My brain felt like it had been plugged into a socket, a spigot turned on in my nose, and the nausea peaked. I was finally able to eject some, but not all, of the contents of my stomach.

Minutes later, Brandy half carried me—still clutching my bucket—to an adjacent room and helped me onto a heated massage table. The session was over. Having purified my system, I was now supposed to rest. I was supposed to feel mildly euphoric now that the suffering was over. But suffering and bile were still very much in me, and resting comfortably was not an option.

On the massage table, I posted myself up on all fours. Head over the bucket, throat raw, tissue dingleberries on my stubble, I wondered: Was it worth the agony?

Given the alternative, it was.

THE COURAGEOUS COWARD

In nearly two decades working for ABC News, I've cultivated the image of a reporter who emerges from the wreckage of a disaster with the story, and casually flicks off the dust. A connoisseur of the close scrape, I've nearly had my foot blown off in Afghanistan, raced through sniper fire in Lebanon, and been the captive of Venezuela's secret police for five days. I've swum with anacondas in the Amazon and tiger sharks in the Bahamas, been in a tornado's "bear cage" and the eyes of hurricanes.

That public persona of jovial fearlessness has obscured a secret, twenty-plus-year battle with panic disorder. Just as an orgasm is the maximal expression of physical pleasure, a panic attack is the maximal expression of anxiety. Though the cocktail of symptoms and possible triggers a panicker might face are as unique as a fingerprint, panic is typically defined as a spasm of debilitating fear in the absence of real danger. And like an orgasm, panic is a disorienting explosion of sensation that could leave you sweaty, panting, and foggy-brained.

My panics are triggered by the bread and butter of my job as a TV reporter: presenting on live television. A live report typically entails speaking for fifteen to forty seconds—anywhere from twenty-five to seventy-five words, or roughly the number of words you've just read in this paragraph. This would not seem particularly taxing. But try regurgitating those twenty-five or so words during a panic, with your heart rattling against your rib cage and a demonic gremlin with a pot of Wite-Out erasing your memory of how to breathe, much less talk.

Millions of viewers have watched my brain short-circuit on their screens. The vast majority wouldn't have registered it as a choke. On my side of the camera, I feel like an adrenalized drunk, stumbling away from the bar, using every fiber of my being just not to fall down. In the days that followed an on-air panic, I would nurse a shame hangover, belittling myself for a C+ performance, and ask a recurring question: What the hell is wrong with me? Am I the product of some malevolent kink in the genetic code?

The irony is that, in my line of work, I confront plenty of *real* (physical) danger. In that sense, I embody a paradox: the courageous coward. When inserted into real-world chaos and peril, I soar. When expected to perform in the calm of a live shot, I crash. One of the hallmarks of panic disorder is the fear of losing control. Long before I knew that, I was dogged by the fear that in a panic I'd either blurt out the wrong thing or nothing at all. You can't edit a live report. There is no taking it back. And once something is broadcast, it spawns on the internet, where it lives in perpetuity.

So why was it, I wondered, that I lacked the fear of great

bodily harm but brimmed with the fear of great reputational harm? Why not the other way around?

A TV reporter whose biggest fear is presenting a live report is like a free solo climber afraid of heights. So I obsessively covered up my Achilles' heel from friends and colleagues. I even kept it from myself. When I'd mention these brain blackouts in my journals, I'd do it cryptically, scribbling entries in shorthand that even I could barely decipher.

It took me years to recognize that what I had long dismissed as "just nerves" were in fact symptoms of panic disorder. It was only in recent years that I began addressing the problem in earnest with a new psychiatrist—even as I remained oblivious to the full extent of the shadow that panic cast over me. We tried everything from antidepressants to ADHD medications, from benzos like Xanax to antiseizure medication. I regularly practiced mindfulness and meditation. I ate well and exercised.

My panic vanquished them all.

Still, through it all, my facade of imperturbability remained plastered in place. This required some sleight of hand: meditation masked as napping (this was when meditation was still considered fringe); the popping of a pill cloaked in a cough; gulping air like a free diver in the minute before a live report to avoid hypoxia on camera. I developed a series of pre–live shot rituals that included push-ups and, sometimes, cigarettes. I indulged in magical thinking. There were a couple of "lucky" pairs of underwear in rotation, which I bought in Paris in 2015 during my coverage of the terrorist attacks there. On that particular tragedy, and the chaotic hunt for the terrorist cell responsible, it seemed the news gods had graced me with near-miraculous luck and poise—which for some reason I attributed to the cheesy 3D-patterned boxer briefs. Throughout, I recognized how silly my one-man panic theater was. I'd shake my head, chuckle to myself—and then return to my regularly scheduled superstition.

Perhaps in anointing a pair of underwear "panic-resistant," I was alone. But unfortunately, there is a lot of company in my misery. More than a quarter of all Americans will suffer a panic attack in their lifetime. That's at least eighty-five million hyperventilating, palpitating people. Some panic experts believe the real number could be closer to 50 percent of Americans. In the years since I began researching this book, hundreds of people have confided in me about their panics—people who would never admit it, even in an anonymous survey. The CEO whose panic stalks him in the dead of night; the college thespian whose terror is provoked by the prospect of a chat with a supermarket cashier; the travel agent so certain he was dying of cardiac arrest that he voiced a goodbye message to his wife and kids. That's to say nothing of those for whom the fear of panic is so pervasive they can no longer step outside their homes.

The sad fact is that the rate of recovery for panic disorder is low, relapse is high, and, shockingly, the severity of disability and dysfunction is higher than that of alcohol dependence. Most of those who suffer from panic have a high baseline of anxiety. We carry around baggage, in other words. For some of us, the baggage is so heavy that the brain considers any added weight of stress a mortal threat. In such cases it pulls the body's fire alarm: a panic attack.

There is no known "cure" for panic. While it can be treated—sometimes easily—it is also unpredictable, which both increases the torment and lulls you into the false belief of its impermanence. It begets more superstition: *Maybe that last formula (Xanax + push-ups + lucky underwear + deep breathing + cigarette) did the trick. I finally beat panic!*

And then, *bam*. It's back.

The most common root cause of panic attacks is social—the fear of judgment and scrutiny by others. Unfortunately for so many of us, this Covid-19-dominated part of the decade has forced humans simultaneously into periodic isolation and more frequent performative interactions. As Dr. Randy Nesse of Arizona State University, one of the founders of evolutionary psychiatry, puts it, for the first time in human history the reign of social media has created "huge competition for perfect performances before huge audiences. There was nothing like it in the Paleolithic," back when we lived in small cave groups and a PowerPoint was merely what you did upon spotting a mammoth.

For many, even their home is no longer a refuge from the threat of constant assessment. Where a phone call once sufficed, the video technology of Zoom, FaceTime, and WhatsApp requires ever greater presentability. We fret not only about our faces and hair, but what our screen backgrounds say about us.

The incidence of panic in the United States and worldwide is so difficult to pin down partly because the majority of people suffering from it don't know what has hit them. Panic attacks so convincingly mimic heart attacks that a third of all patients presenting at emergency rooms for cardiac events are actually suffering from panic. That means that over 2.5 million Americans rush to a hospital each year thinking they could be dying of heart failure, when in fact their hearts are perfectly fine. "They breathe really shallow or really fast, feel sweaty, feel tightness in the chest, complain of numbness," says Kelly Kropholler, a retired emergency dispatcher. In seventeen years under the headset, she answered hundreds of 911 calls for both panic attacks and heart attacks. Even Kropholler's practiced ear often couldn't tell the difference. "All of those physical symptoms of [peak] anxiety present as a heart attack clinically," she said.

Diagnoses, both psychological and physiological, are squishy because, in many respects, science is still in the Stone Age when it comes to understanding the three pounds of electric Jell-O inside our skull. At the time of this writing, the most sophisticated animal brain mapped is that of the lowly fruit fly—which has about 860,000 times fewer neurons than the human brain. Even if we could map the human brain, it would only provide us with a blueprint to an incomprehensibly complex system—like a user's manual for an alien spacecraft written in alien. In the meantime, psychologists, psychiatrists, and neurologists continue to debate why we suffer maladies like anxiety and panic, and why some medications like antidepressants work for only some of the people some of the time.

We do know that when it comes to mental illness, nearly everyone has *something*, or is close to someone who does. According to the Centers for Disease Control and Prevention, more than half of Americans will be diagnosed with a mental disorder at some point in their lifetime. Many suffer without the clarity of a diagnosis. The human brain is a marvel of multitasking, processing computations like a supercomputer while humming along on a frugal twenty watts of energy—the equivalent of one of those dim nightstand lightbulbs. But every once in a while, even this marvel suffers a "blue screen of death," a fatal error in its code that crashes the whole system. The moments between the crash and the reboot—the throes of peak panic—can be terrifying. And as I've learned, they can also be ruinous.

THIS BOOK?

In bed, as I read yet another book on the human body and anxiety, my wife, Daphna, leaned over and touched my arm. "What do you think the end is going to be?"

"Of *this* book?" I nodded to the one in my hands.

"No, the book *you're* writing."

"Oh," I responded.

She continued, "Is the protagonist going to be cured?"

For most of my journey into the heart of panic, I had no answer to that question. My wife's protagonist walked down a long corridor, checking every door for relief, unsure what relief would even look like, much less which door to try. Over nearly four years, I turned the handle of almost every door I could find: from the ground truth of evolutionary science to psychologists to psychics (not helpful) to psychedelics (very helpful).*

I reached for the most convenient door first: pharmacology. Of the limitless smorgasbord of pills on the market, I reasoned, there must be some recipe of chemicals that can cure panic. Surely my shrink, with his magical prescription pad, could conjure up something for me.

I've tried. From experience, I can tell you that recipe does not exist.

If I couldn't grasp exactly why my brain short-circuited when it did, perhaps I could better understand the biological mechanisms of panic more broadly. I boned up on the hormonal cascade called the stress response, which you might know as the fight-or-flight response. It's an ideal system for hightailing it from a saber-toothed tiger and is still crucial for

---

* I spent a lot of money on a two-hour session with a big-name psychic. She was very nice but not very accurate.

the survival of our species. It's less useful if it kicks in when you're standing safely in front of a camera trying to spit out a few ungarbled words.

Eventually, I would learn that my body's stress response, though achingly disruptive, was not wrong, exactly. Evolutionary biologists and psychologists showed me the beauty of that chemical orchestra and the precision with which each body marches to its beat. They taught me that our brain is not actually designed for us to be "happy" or even content most of the time. It is designed foremost to keep us alive. In that sense, there was relief in the knowledge that my body was working just as engineered—even *during* a panic.

In those conversations with evolutionary psychologists, I learned why our "unreasonable" social anxiety is actually *totally* reasonable and how psychology has been invalidating fears that, evolutionarily, are quite valid. That knowledge helped loosen shame's half nelson over my psyche. So I began to flirt with disclosure, first confessing my panic to a total stranger and later to friends and colleagues. After a while I found myself bringing it up in casual conversation. Removing the stain of secrecy, which afflicts so many of us, proved a comforting balm. Panic still seemed to carry the stigma that other diagnoses, like anxiety and depression, no longer did. As the chief medical officer of the American Psychological Association put it to me, even just by "coming out" publicly with panic, I could help put a dent in that stigma.

Since modern science and conventional therapy seemed unable to provide a cure, I gravitated toward the more unconventional. I became a human laboratory experiment. There was hypnosis and seismically cathartic experiences while doing breathwork. That led me to another space that scientists are studying in earnest: psychedelics. In molecules derived from Sonoran toads, Amazonian vines, and Andean cacti, I had my soul, mind, and very often guts wrenched, each time recalibrating my relationship with my psyche.

When I mentioned these experiences to others, people would routinely smirk, maybe envisioning *Fear and Loathing in Las Vegas,* with Johnny Depp slaloming across Vegas in a convertible Chevy Caprice. As you'll see, these were no drug-fueled joyrides. Some were pure, uncut misery. And my ride in each instance was a couch or a bed, with a facilitator or a clinical psychiatrist riding shotgun. Taken together, they allowed me to see, better than any conventional therapy I'd tried, that, for me, panic was a presenting symptom—that there were other parts of me that screamed for healing.

Eventually I found that healing. It came in the form of emotional surrender, which occasionally yielded cloudbursts of catharsis. These were marathon sobbing sessions—bigger, uglier, and more numerous than I had thought possible.

My journey was neither planned out in advance nor scientifically conducted. My path was not direct, and it was definitely not replicable. Parts of it are not particularly advisable. I made a bunch of sometimes comically wrong turns. (Please feel free to laugh when you encounter them.) I also hit dead ends. But I hope that my circuitous road trip toward healing helps you, or someone you care about, find your own more direct route toward a truce with your mind.

A cottage industry of books promises methods that stop panic "instantly" with one recently discovered Amazonian miracle remedy or a dozen "easy-to-remember" techniques. I dearly hope those work for you. They did not work for me. A one-size-fits-all solution to panic does not exist—if it did, I wouldn't have felt compelled to write this book.

But I'm confident that, if you or your loved ones have lived with panic attacks as I have, you'll find comfort, and practical solutions, in the pages that follow.

Panic is not easy to conquer or even manage. It can sometimes feel like medieval punishment. But it doesn't have to be a life sentence.

DOOMSDAY CLOCK

Every year since 1947, the Bulletin of Atomic Scientists has updated its "Doomsday Clock," a metaphor for how close humanity is to destroying itself. At its founding, the Bulletin's now-iconic clock was set at seven minutes to midnight. At the time of this writing, due to the war in Ukraine and the ravages of climate change, the clock is set at ninety seconds to midnight—the closest we've been to self-annihilation, in the scientists' estimation, since 1953, when nuclear powers would use Pacific atolls for atomic target practice.

For a big chunk of my adult life, my mental "Doomsday Clock" was set at, let's say, 120 seconds to midnight—just two minutes away from a chain reaction of anxiety that would trigger a panic-driven meltdown of the mind. When the mushroom cloud cleared, I'd be professionally and personally radioactive, shedding failure isotopes wherever I went.

Like those atomic scientists, I had a solid idea of what might trigger my Armageddon—an ill-timed, crippling panic attack, of course—but little sense of the specific circumstances that might bring it about. As it turned out, it wouldn't be in any of the hair-raising places my work had previously taken me but close to home, literally and emotionally.

For me, the clock struck midnight on the misty morning of January 26, 2020, during a live special report on the crash that killed forty-one-year-old Kobe Bryant, his thirteen-year-old daughter Gianna, and seven others. Having suffered hundreds of similar episodes over the previous twenty years, I instantly diagnosed what had commandeered my brain as

I delivered my report: a full-on panic. But unlike any panic before or since, this one caused me to make a fundamental journalistic error.

Out of sensitivity to the Bryant family and their loss, I won't replay the details here. They've suffered enough, and my tiny role in their story can be only an unfortunate footnote to a heartbreaking tragedy. Suffice to say it was the worst mistake I'd ever committed as a reporter, and the shame of it has dogged me since.

For years I'd felt the hot breath of a reckoning on the back of my neck. I imagined I risked professional collapse with each live shot. Sustaining the appearance of the never-ruffled TV persona threatened my emotional collapse. It left me fantasizing about living panic-free—a life that had long seemed incompatible with my job as an on-air correspondent.

But in the aftermath of that January morning, there was no longer a choice: I had to either leave TV news or resolve my panic.

Eventually, there would be a resolution—but not yet, not nearly. On that January morning, standing on a mist-shrouded hillside, my first step would be to deliver an on-air correction and an apology to ABC's viewers. Our crew had staked out a position on the sidewalk. A crescent of onlookers formed around our cameraman. I was looking at the lens; they were looking at me.

As I delivered my apology, I recognized a face among them. It was a mother who had trick-or-treated at my house with her two daughters on Halloween. We had clicked over a conversation that ranged from costumes and candy to her holistic medical practice. Now, three months later, she eyed me with a mixture of horror, disgust, and pity.

I knew that look.

CHAPTER 1

Textbook Panic

t was 1990, and I reached out a fat-dimpled hand to the mourners at Temple Emanu-El Synagogue in Westfield, New Jersey. I was twelve, and pleasantly stoned on a combo of shock and the Xanax our doctor had doled out to the entire family. Outside the synagogue, cars gridlocked the parking lot. Inside, mourners were stacked all the way to the brass nameplates on the back wall memorializing the dead.

My mother, sister, and I stood near the pulpit in the front. From our position, I observed with glazed eyes the lengthening line to offer condolences. I gamely fielded well-intentioned comments about the turnout—seen by some as a benchmark of a lifetime's achievement. Many remarked that my dad, with his lopsided grin, was just so easy to like. *Charming* was the word they used. One business associate guffawed, "I'll never forget when he came into our business meeting . . . *walking on his hands!*"

A born pleaser, I gamely returned their sad smiles and offerings of comfort. Playing to the refrain I heard often that day—that I was now "the man of the house"—I made what felt like adult pronouncements. A bunch of times I trotted out a line I'd overheard grown-ups use about other people who'd passed, delivered in a voice, at twelve, still cartoonishly squeaky.

"Well, at least he'd lived a full life."

My father had been forty-two when the Cessna in which he'd been a passenger plummeted out of the Georgia sky on a bluebird September morning in 1990. My pronouncements were met with a look of eye-popping anguish mixed with shock and a dash of horror. The look would be seared into my memory. I would think of it as the "you poor fucking kid" face.

Thirty years later, in December 2019, I turned forty-two myself and, over the next couple of months, grappled with the weirdness of outliving my father. I had always assumed forty-two would be the natural terminus of my life, if I even made it that far. It didn't make life more depressing—it made it more urgent. To prepare for that eventuality, I'd spent years racking up life experiences like merit badges: love at first sight in Buenos Aires, war in the Middle East, wedding on a Tel Aviv beach, jail in Latin America, children, mortgage, dog, a submarine ride to the bottom of the ocean. It was enough living to have satisfied the "full life" I mentioned to those mourners at my dad's funeral.

Some friends had wondered if I'd even *courted* an early exit. During seven years in the Middle East in my twenties, I had taken some moronic risks reporting from war-torn Iraq, Afghanistan, Syria, Lebanon, and Gaza—though my "moronic" risks were still a step down from the "suicidal" risks taken by some colleagues. Marriage and two children ended the most extreme risk-taking, but not the urge to be where life is closest to death—zones of catastrophe wrought by man or nature. Reporting from the edge also meant becoming the reporter who could reliably elicit emotion from an interviewee. I achieved that by speaking in our common language of loss, which required making myself vulnerable—essentially becoming a receptacle for other people's pain. You might call it emotional recklessness.

Those years of living in full coincided neatly with the dawn of my age of panic. My twenty-year ascent from print to radio to TV journalist was accompanied by a rising crescendo of panic attacks, one that reached its inevitable denouement that January morning in 2020, a day that was tragic for so many Angelenos but that carried with it for me an air of finality.

As I issued my correction and wrapped up my live shot, there was no panic—just typical nerves spiked with the rotgut of shame. I may have offered an accidental window into my psyche when I referred over my shoulder to "that plane" (not helicopter). Over the next couple of hours, our team remained busy with preparing for the next broadcasts, including an instant one-hour *20/20* special, for which I had the lead story. There was little time for rumination. There would be plenty of that to come later.

At some point in those hazy hours, I was informed that after the *20/20* special I would be permanently removed from further coverage of the story. The hammer was dropping.

THE CURSE OF THE DEVIL

The *Diagnostic and Statistical Manual of Mental Disorders,* or *DSM,* the nearly thousand-page handbook psychiatrists use to diagnose mental illnesses, defines a panic attack as "an abrupt surge of intense fear or intense discomfort that reaches a peak within minutes." In that time, a pupu platter of unpleasant symptoms might occur, including but not limited to: heart palpitations, sweating, trembling, shortness of breath, chest pain, nausea, dizziness, and feelings of unreality. Many other definitions, like the one from the Mayo Clinic, qualify that symptoms occur "when there is no real danger or apparent cause."

Fear helps us survive in the present moment. Imagine you're standing on railroad tracks and you notice a train bearing down on you. But your foot is caught under a railroad tie. Your racing heart and trembling aren't symptoms of a panic attack; they're just plain old terror, because your life is threatened. Your body is mounting a response that can help get your foot unstuck and the rest of your body off the tracks alive. What is not considered a "real danger": freaking out in the same way because you're about to go on air or talk on a Zoom or drive in a tunnel. That is a "perceived" threat of something bad happening in an undetermined future moment, and thus deemed the trigger for a panic attack. (Although, as we'll see, perceived threats might be far more real than the *DSM* gives them credit for.)

Dr. Michael Telch, the founding director of the University of Texas Laboratory for the Study of Anxiety Disorders, says the peak of panic is generally short-lived, lasting less than a minute. "Panic is really the period of the assessment of danger," Telch explains. For those who suffer from panic, nearly anything can trigger it: the physical sensation of an apple seed stuck in your throat; a smell that evokes past trauma; a feared reduction in your ability to breathe (like when you're in a packed elevator); and, often, a social cue.

Panic often manifests out of the blue. Like the spectral Dementors in the Harry Potter series, panics can descend in swarms, strangling you with invisible hands and sucking the air out of your lungs. Also like the Dementors, they seem to arrive at the most inopportune times. And anyone who has suffered a panic attack can tell you that where there's panic, there's shame, trailing it like body odor.

Panic disorder, which about 5 percent of Americans will experience in their lifetime, is defined as unexpected and repeated episodes of peak fear, coupled with chronic anxiety about having panic. Telch believes the disorder is massively underdiagnosed. That's because, he says, a real diagnosis for panic disorder doesn't even require frequent panics, or even *a single panic in a decade,* so long as a patient feels a persistent and potent fear of having one. It's a disorder predicated on the fear of fear. For many of the dozens of panickers I've spoken to in researching this book, that dread of a future panic is debilitating precisely because it seems ever present, always lurking just around the corner for the next sneak attack.

Panickers will often report their panics last for "hours." But Telch and other mental health professionals say that once that initial period of threat assessment is over—anywhere from fifteen to sixty seconds—the actual clinical panic ends. What's left is a heightened state of anxiety, which is awful but more manageable: anxiety is a condition that, to varying degrees, all of us cope with daily.

The single most common root cause of panic attacks is glossophobia, the fear of public speaking. It is so pervasive that three out of four people are said to experience it in their lifetime. The National Institute of Mental Health classifies glossophobia as the most common subset of the most common phobia: social phobia.

It's not only stereotypically nervous people who experience panic from social anxiety. I am uncommonly gregarious; my near-compulsion to talk to strangers, to find common ground with nearly every person I meet, has yielded enduring friendships, journalistic mini-scoops, and frequent embarrassment for my children. I'm not just socially fearless; ever since taking headers out of my crib and toddling across the street to neighbors' homes, I have lived most of my life with an extremely high tolerance for physical fear. A tempered version of this has persisted into my mid-forties.

But I have learned to be terrified of panic.

A panic attack is one of the few psychological phenomena that make many sufferers feel *certain* they are going to die. If it seems like this fear resides solely in a panic attack sufferer's head, it doesn't—though it does start there. As neuropsychologist Justin Feinstein explains, panic attacks are your brain and body telling you that "if you don't resolve these [perceived] threats immediately you could potentially die. It feels as real as if you were having a heart attack, or as if you were suffocating."

When Feinstein was doing his clinical internship at a VA hospital, he recalls, one patient turned up in the emergency room nearly every week for a year. "And we asked the most obvious questions," Feinstein says. " 'Don't you realize that there's really nothing wrong with you physically? That you're okay?' And they go: 'Yes, yes, I get it. I cognitively understand it. But in the moment of a panic attack, all that rationale goes out the door. I feel like I'm really dying.' "

It's easy to think of this individual as an outlier, an extreme version of your run-of-the-mill panic sufferer. Unfortunately, that is not the case. In 2018, doctors from Indiana University's Department of Emergency Medicine surveyed over four hundred emergency departments in forty-six states about their treatment of patients for cardiac arrest. The data showed something shocking: about one in three "cardiac" patients was having a panic or anxiety attack, not a heart attack. Since heart disease kills nearly 700,000 Americans annually—more than any other disease—doctors did their due diligence putting these patients through a battery of cardiac tests, sometimes lasting days, and costing many thousands of dollars. Even then, doctors found nothing wrong with those patients' hearts.[*]

According to CDC data from 2019, more than eight million patients annually show up at emergency departments with chest pain. That could mean more than 2.6 million people a year with perfectly functional hearts present at ERs with phantom heart attacks. One study sponsored by the federal government's Agency for Healthcare Research and Quality estimates that the potential cost of undiagnosed panic to our health care system likely runs to the billions. Just from the all-too-common misdiagnosis of panic.

You might be among those millions of patients. If you aren't, I wouldn't fault you for thinking that these would-be heart attack sufferers are just hypochondriacs. But as Kelly Kropholler, the veteran 911 dispatcher, observes, panic attack patients are "diuretic, they're sweaty, they're breathing really shallow or really fast, and they have tightness in their chest. They complain of numbness." Anyone who has watched TV over the past few decades has learned enough to instantly recognize these symptoms as evidence of a heart attack. And if your panic disorder is undiagnosed (or if you are suffering a panic attack for the first time), these chest-clutching, disorienting, hyperventilating experiences almost perfectly mimic an honest-to-god heart attack.

"Panic" covers a wide range of symptoms, and estimates of the total number of Americans afflicted with panic attacks (rather than panic disorder specifically) are all over the map. A 2006 Harvard meta-survey found that 28 percent of American respondents meet the criteria for suffer-

---

[*] Further, 58 percent of all people who presented at emergency rooms with chest pain had anxiety or panic disorders as a contributing factor.

ing a panic attack in their lifetime—over eighty-five million people, or more than the population of Germany. From his forty years of studying panic, UT's Michael Telch estimates the real number is about double that. He believes around half of all Americans have suffered or will suffer a panic attack in their lifetime—whether they know it or not. And if you have suffered trauma—clinically defined as exposure to actual or threatened death, serious injury, or sexual violence—you are far more likely to have a panic attack in your lifetime.

Surveys consistently find that twice as many women suffer from panic disorder as men. It is impossible to say whether the greater rate of women with panic reflects a greater incidence or whether women are more likely to self-report their panic disorder than men. Anecdotally, I can tell you that over the past couple of years, in describing this book to male friends or acquaintances, many of them have confided that they, too, suffer panic attacks but keep them secret. Anxiety specialists tell me it may also be that men have higher rates of alcoholism and drug abuse than women, which they use to self-medicate and numb a variety of mental health issues. Either way, regardless of gender, most of those afflicted with panic do their suffering in silence.

Very often that's because panic sufferers have no idea what's hit them. According to that Indiana University study of emergency department visits, almost two-thirds of the patients who erroneously thought they were having a heart attack *were not informed* by treating physicians at the hospital that this was a panic attack and *not* a heart attack. Why? The study found that hospital staff often felt their hospital's mental health resources lacking and they were uncomfortable giving psychological diagnoses when their expertise is physiological—a patient's body, not mind.

Let's digest all that data for a minute. It suggests that

untold numbers of patients might continue to believe, erroneously, that their hearts are the problem and that they are a hair's breadth from possible death. Equally tragic, says evolutionary psychiatrist Randy Nesse, who spent years working in the emergency room, is what he calls the *semi*-diagnosis. That's when an ER doctor tells a patient, "I don't think it is your heart, but come back fast if it happens again." A message intended to encourage healthy monitoring, it can instead become a "small symptom escalating to a big attack," says Nesse. In other words, *"come back fast"* turns into a call for hypervigilance toward the patient's (nonexistent) heart condition or, even worse, another nonexistent mystery condition. With just such a push, a one-off panic might easily escalate into something recurring—including full-blown panic disorder.

Panic can strike in all sorts of ways, at all different times. For most people, however, panic begins to attack in the late teens or early twenties. In that respect, my first full-throated, knock-your-socks-off panic arrived right on cue.

A THESIS IN PANIC

I had applied to college as the new millennium approached. The Iron Curtain had fallen, a surge of high-tech prosperity had arisen, and the world seemed drunk on optimism. Editors rolled out magazine covers like the one from a 1997 issue of *Wired* that my stepfather brought home for us to marvel at: "The Long Boom: A History of the Future, 1980–2020." It proclaimed: "We're facing 25 years of prosperity, freedom, and a better environment for the whole world. You got a problem with that?"*

---

* Turns out neither *Wired* magazine nor I was very good at prophecy.

My family certainly did not.

You may have heard it said that Jewish mothers want their children to grow up to be doctors or lawyers or accountants. That was so twentieth century. Looking toward the new millennium, my mother would say: "You could be a prophet." It was always said half in jest from an adoring mother, and it came despite my strenuous efforts to disabuse her of the notion by peppering my general high achievement with acts of teenage self-sabotage.

Her vision of a prophet-son was not religious. I was to be a supercharged activist for social justice, a young man who would single-mindedly battle oppression, abuse, and corruption. The crown jewel of my application to Williams College, in the frigid northwest corner of Massachusetts, was my personal essay, which shamelessly exploited my mother's filial aspirations. It started with much winking about my mother's lofty goals for her son (jokes my mom was in on), then asking playfully: *Can I major in prophesy? Do they offer "prophet" courses at Williams?*

Prophet or not, the essay seems to have won the intended yuks; the school admitted me. As for its effect on me, no matter the love with which the message was delivered, I internalized the maternal anointment as an admonishment: It's not enough to be good; you need to be damned near perfect.

If that essay was my first academic exercise at Williams, my last came on a crisp evening in May 2000. I was giving an informal oral presentation of my senior thesis in political science, which I had spent the previous nine months researching and writing. But instead of a summation of my two-hundred-page dissertation on Turkish-Israeli relations, what I delivered for my audience was a textbook panic attack.

At some point in the fifteen seconds between when the

poli-sci chair announced my name and when he ended his brief description of my thesis, my heart had begun to jack-hammer. It was as if I'd launched into a dead sprint just sitting in my chair. My teeth felt like they were loosening from my jaw—that rinse of fear you get when a cop pulls you over. Dutifully, my feet carried the rest of me to the lectern, which I white-knuckled to avoid falling through the floor.

Assembled before me were my esteemed professors and fellow political science majors, all of whom I suspected were as brilliant as I was average. There were probably a few dozen people in the room, though I couldn't see them. My vision had constricted to a pinhole. I knew they were waiting for me to speak, but the turtleneck that I had selected for the occasion, so perfectly intellectual in appearance, now felt like a pack of feral cats clawing at my throat.

I struggled to form words. I have no idea how long I hovered up there; it was either very short or very long. I am confident, however, that all of them thought I was a blithering idiot. I had amassed a mountain of knowledge about Turkish-Israeli relations in the preceding months, but scanning my brain I found just a few piles of dust. I tried to sound casual, but my voice was reedy and strained. Words must have come out of my mouth, but they were heavy and tasted like sand. I was standing stock-still, but I couldn't catch my breath.

If clinicians define a panic attack as a spasm of debilitating fear in the absence of real danger, then that night twenty-some years ago would seem to fit the bill precisely. I knew everyone in the room (one was my best friend). There were no academic consequences for a flop, because the talk wasn't graded. Hell, it wasn't even required!

Somehow I wrapped up my presentation. Loosening my grip on the podium, I sloshed back into my chair alongside the other students. I stared straight ahead, trying to act like nothing had happened, hoping the flop-sweat slicking my body hadn't soaked through my clothes.

If you had asked me then, I wouldn't have even been aware that I suffered from *anxiety*, let alone panic. (And I was even going to therapy at the time!) Depression was a thing people talked about then, anxiety much less so. Besides, I thought: there's no way I had anxiety—I was an outgoing achiever.

I could tell, however, that it was something bigger than everyday butterflies. It would take well over a decade for me to learn that in the college hall that evening, though it felt like I was molting into a werewolf, something else had possessed my body.

FIGHT, FLIGHT, OR FREEZE

Unless you're dozing, you're processing the words you're reading right now with the front part of your brain, called the frontal lobe. That lobe houses the prefrontal cortex, a region of the brain in charge of higher cognitive function: processes like problem solving, critical thinking, focusing on a task, and curbing impulses. It's the kind of brain activity that makes everyday reasoning, sudoku, and fantasy football possible. A different, less evolved part of your brain is charged with sensing danger and initiating your fight-or-flight response. It's called the amygdala. In the instant my name was announced that spring night in 2000, even before my thinking brain had had a chance to react, the amygdala, a pair of almond-shaped nerve bundles, started buzzing.

Evolutionarily speaking, the amygdala is among the oldest parts of our brain. You actually have two amygdalae, one in each cerebral hemisphere, but scientists tend to refer to them in the singular. The amygdala sits in deep center field of your brain, behind your eyes—in position to catch incoming sensory stimuli, whether from your vision, hearing, smell, touch, or taste. Some psychologists and neurologists liken the amygdala to our innate "smoke detectors." If the system it belongs to fails, you could miss a key sensory input—like, say, the ten-car pileup unfolding in front of you on the interstate—with fatal consequences.

In good times, the frontal cortex and amygdala complement each other like a buddy cop duo. The amygdala is nervous by design, sensing danger everywhere; it's constantly pulling fire alarms. The more restrained frontal cortex regulates that reaction, basically calling off the fire department and assuring them that actually everything is just fine. But during times of stress, the frontal cortex's influence over the amygdala weakens and the impulsive amygdala gains the upper hand—going full crazy-eyes Mel Gibson from *Lethal Weapon*. That's when the brain's command center, the hypothalamus, jumps into action.

The hypothalamus is a marble-sized node located just above the brain stem. This is yet another ancient part of our brain, which acts like a thermostat for our hormones, maintaining the homeostasis (balance) of processes including sex drive, temperature control, hunger and thirst, circadian rhythm, emotional expression, and blood pressure. Because the amygdala and the hypothalamus have had this key role in animals' brains for hundreds of millions of years, the system they belong to is commonly referred to as our reptilian brain.

The hypothalamus manages tactical operations. It sends distress signals to the pituitary glands, which in turn fire off signals to the little nodes atop our kidneys called the adrenal glands. The adrenals secrete a chemical messenger that engages our survival reflexes, leaving us ready to take defensive or offensive action. That chemical messenger is epinephrine, which you likely know as adrenaline.

All of this sensing and signaling, the recruitment and deployment of our body's hormonal Navy SEALs, happens in a fraction of a second. So back in college, when I was called to the podium to speak, adrenaline had begun spurting into my system before my thinking brain had registered any chemical change whatsoever.*

The activation of the acute stress response prepared my body to flee, fight, or freeze.† The impulse to fight is characterized by clenched teeth, tightened fists, angry stares, and sometimes homicidal thoughts. Flight is all restlessness, feeling trapped, shallow breath, and thoughts of doom. The third part of that stress response, freezing, is less discussed but equally fascinating. In freezing, the heart rate slows, as does breathing. A person might feel trapped in their body, or numb and cold. Freezing happens when the brain tells the body that the options to flee or fight are unavailable.

One form of freezing is called tonic immobility—basically, fainting. You've likely seen it yourself, certainly in the movies. In humans it can be triggered when a person sees blood, a syringe, or a skin-breaking wound (or their wife giving birth), then faints. This is called an extreme stress survival response, which evolved with the rise of intraspecies violence—when humans turned murderous during the Paleolithic period. If

---

* New studies suggest that a panic attack can often begin up to an hour *before* the onset of full-blown symptoms. So it's quite possible that I was breathing more heavily, taking in more oxygen, and depleting my carbon dioxide while still in my dorm or at dinner in the cafeteria.

† Some researchers also include faint and fawn. You've likely noticed fawning in dogs. After they poop on your favorite rug, they'll hunch submissively, look up at you with big eyes, and wag their tail in rapid and short swings, ingratiating themselves. Humans, too, exhibit ingratiating behaviors.

a person had no options to fight or flee, their death seemingly inescapable, an ability to convincingly play dead could save their life. Those survivors ensured that fainting became embedded into our genome.*

Fainting might have only reduced my misery that night. My body was in full flight mode instead, with nowhere to go. My adrenaline surged. On the savannah, that would confer obvious advantages. When a lion bursts out of the brush, adrenaline pumps oxygen and glucose to the muscles in our arms and legs, ensuring our ability to run fast, and to keep running even after the lion has taken a bite out of our ass. My pupils dilated (likely because our ancestors were most vulnerable at night) and my senses sharpened—specifically, my smell, hearing, and vision, as well as my brain's internal GPS. I began to sweat (one argument for sweating during panic is that it made early humans more slippery and harder to catch).

But as we've seen, the stress response also inhibits our ability to draw from our long-term memory. This makes sense; when a lion is chasing you, there are more important things to think about than, say, when you last called your mother. That may be why during that college talk my skull felt like it was stuffed with cotton candy and why remembering basic facts stored in my brain for years, like the capital of Turkey, proved impossible.

To keep itself primed for action, the body dispatches the

---

* Dr. Temple Grandin, acclaimed animal behaviorist and the author of *Animals in Translation,* says that when chickens, some breeds of goats, and zebus (a subspecies of African cow), among other species, encounter certain threats, they also go into tonic immobility. Grandin explains that when you're slow, clumsy, and squawky—like a chicken—sometimes appearing as close to dead as possible might keep you from being eaten. The complete lack of movement and subdued breathing just might make the animal invisible to a predator. Certain breeds of goats are the stars of the massive "fainting goats" subgenre on YouTube.

hormone cortisol, whose job it is to muster the necessary energy to *continue* to fight or flee.* To ensure sufficient energy reserves, cortisol musters the suspension of "nonessential" functions: digestion, long-term memory, sex drive, parts of the immune system. That explains my parched mouth that night in college; salivation is a part of our digestive system. With digestion temporarily suspended, my bowels also loosened. In practical terms, because squeezing liquid from the contents of our intestines uses a lot of energy that would be better used running away, my colon was trying to quickly get rid of my cafeteria dinner.†

Suffice it to say that, apart from what I actually said during my talk—which, mercifully, I'll never know—it was a memorable night.

A SHORT HISTORY OF PANIC

Many evolutionary milestones, like the first murder, the first joke, or the first panic attack, are lost to time. But it's fair to guess that panic has been a human companion for as long as human civilization has been around. One of the first recorded references to it came nearly 2,000 years ago, in the writings of the Greek philosopher Plutarch. "There hapned in the night a sudden feare and fright among them without any apparant cause, such as they call Panique Frights," goes one 1603 English translation, "wherewith being woonder-

---

* Or, more commonly, to exercise.
† Your colon typically takes its time reabsorbing liquid as you digest food, but when cortisol is activated and digestion is suspended, it expedites that process. This is why loose bowels and diarrhea plague people with anxiety and panic. Gazelles and deer poop in fright before they take flight—animals are faster after dropping a load.

fully troubled and scarred, they went a shipboord, without all order."*

The etymology of the word *panic* derives from the ancient Greek god Pan, the patron of nature and mountains, the consort of many a nymph, and the possessor of a scream so unpleasant it scared off the Titans. Many panickers know that scream implicitly.

The word *panic* came into more common use in the nineteenth century; usage in English evolved from a reference of disorganized retreat to the herd mentality of humans during societal crises. There were the runs on banks that occurred in the face of financial uncertainty, such as in the panics of 1873, 1884, 1890, and 1893. When the 1918 flu pandemic was killing many thousands a week, New York City health commissioner Royal Copeland wrote of wanting "to prevent panic, hysteria, mental disturbance, and thus to protect the public from the conditions of mind that in itself predisposes to physical ills."

Copeland's association of panic with "hysteria" was quite common—a condition historically ascribed to women (the Greek *hystera* means "uterus"). Hysteria suggested not only madness but weakness, a stigma that unfortunately persists. Because the fears that gave rise to such states—whether fears of vomit, spiders, airplane crashes, or public speaking—rarely resulted in harm to the sufferer, the underlying conditions could too easily be written off. They were, it was said, pure hysteria.

Like hysteria, panic has long carried a negative stain. The term was even appropriated in the 1980s by an antigay, antiprogressive coalition in California that called itself the Pre-

---

* Plutarch, *The Philosophie, commonlie called, The Morals*, translated by Philemon Holland (London: Arnold Hatfield, 1603).

vent AIDS Now Initiative Committee, thus PANIC. In 1986, PANIC put forth a ballot measure, Proposition 64, which called for the HIV testing of all Californians and the mass quarantine of the 300,000 people then believed to have been infected with the virus. Californians did the right thing and put a stop to that particular panic; Prop. 64 was voted down 71 to 29 percent in the 1986 California elections.

As for the condition itself, much of the ancient "psychology" around anxiety and panic was influenced by the Greek surgeon, physician, philosopher, and proto-shrink Galen. Among his treatises is *On the Diagnosis and Cure of the Soul's Passion,* a manual on how to coach the afflicted through their "passions," secrets, and fears. Galen was nearly two millennia ahead of his time, calling for what today we would call talk therapy. But unfortunately, that was not to be his great legacy. Instead, Galen would be known for popularizing the theory of the "four humors" that regulate one's passions: black bile, yellow bile, blood, and phlegm. To balance those "humors," Galen developed draining instructions for anything from low mood to a bellyache, which for centuries meant bloodletting, leeches, forced purging, and innumerable patient deaths by "barber surgeons."*

It wasn't until the mid-nineteenth century that the current definition of mental disorders began to take shape. While studying a group of soldiers during the Civil War, the Philadelphia physician Jacob Mendez DaCosta identified a condition comprising both depression and panic. He called it "soldier's heart." Today we call it post-traumatic stress disorder, or

---

* Interestingly, purging is back en vogue big-time. There are a few studies out there urging reconsideration of the potential therapeutic effects of purging, particularly during the use of medicines like ayahuasca.

PTSD. DaCosta's major contribution to our understanding of panic attacks was connecting symptoms of the mind and heart/body into a single ailment that affected both.

After World War II, psychiatrists began clamoring for a systemized classification of the illnesses that seemed to afflict so many of us, from anxiety disorder to schizophrenia. The *Diagnostic and Statistical Manual of Mental Disorders*, or *DSM*—the bible of mental maladies—was born in 1952. At the time, the *DSM*, and psychology in general, was still highly influenced by Sigmund Freud and his work on the unconscious. I'll spare you the tortuous evolution of anxiety nomenclature. Suffice it to say that, for decades, anxiety and panic were classified as forms of "neurosis." Through successive revisions of the *DSM*, those neuroses split off into the conditions whose names we are more familiar with now. It wasn't until 1980 that panic disorder was written into the *DSM* (its third edition) and given its own classification. In the years since, those classifications and the symptoms they describe have been and continue to be further refined.

Neuropsychologist Justin Feinstein says that we are so early in our understanding of the human brain that we still don't know how much we don't know. "I'm guessing it will take another century or so before we have a more detailed understanding of the human brain. In some ways we are still in the Stone Age and in other ways (especially with all the new molecular tools that are being developed, like optogenetics) we are at the beginning of the Renaissance when it comes to neuroscience."

You could say that the dawn of that Stone Age came in the 1960s, when a team led by Nobel laureate Sydney Brenner began to map the wiring of an animal's brain for the first time. They picked the lowly roundworm, which has 302 neurons.

It took Brenner's team decades to complete the task, largely because they had to manually trace all 302 neurons and the thousands of synapses that connect them.

Those brain road maps of neural connections are called connectomes. In late 2021, scientists at the Howard Hughes Medical Institute announced a stunning achievement. They had mapped part of the brain of a creature far more sophisticated than a roundworm: a fruit fly. The fruit fly has about 100,000 neurons—vastly more complex than the roundworm, but also vastly less complex than the human brain, estimated to possess some 86 billion neurons and 100 trillion synapses.[*]

In other words, science may still be fumbling in the dark when it comes to some of the brain's basics. An article published in 2019 by the prestigious Allen Institute for Brain Science outlined the biggest questions about the brain that scientists still face, including how we think, what neurons and brain cells do, and what causes brain disease. If we can't even figure out how humans think, how could we begin to say how billions of neurons interact and, for instance, pop out a panic?

This goes a long way toward explaining our relative ignorance when it comes not just to mental illnesses but to the way we treat them. Says the Allen Institute's Jack Waters: "With drugs like opioids or antidepressants, we actually don't understand the mechanisms of the underlying molecules those drugs are interacting with." Which may be why the efficacy of those drugs is about as reliable as betting on red in roulette: On balance, antidepressants work just a tiny bit better than placebos in the treatment of major depression and anxiety. For many folks with depression, anxiety, and panic,

---

[*] I'm not knocking the fruit fly. Its navigational skills and ability to fly are marvels unrivaled by modern human technology. Heck, even the roundworm may have a few tricks to teach us.

antidepressants don't work at all, yet they come bearing significant side effects and withdrawal symptoms.

A recent survey by the World Health Organization found that people in so-called WEIRD countries—Western, Educated, Industrialized, Rich, and Democratic—report higher rates of anxiety disorder (which includes panic) than people in developing nations. There is a host of possible reasons for that. It could well be that rates of anxiety are lower in developing countries where the social and familial networks critical to people's well-being are stronger than in some of their wealthier neighbors. I'd put my money on that explanation. But it's also possible that, as studies of emergency rooms attest, awareness about panic and related anxiety disorders is simply abysmal in the United States. It may be worse in developing countries.

It could also be that some of the people who have suffered panic attacks, and know it, are ashamed to admit it. Even in anonymous surveys—even to themselves. You might wonder, who are these people so obtuse they don't acknowledge they're suffering a malady that controls their lives? It so happens I know a guy.

CHAPTER 2

Keeping the Secret

I n early 2016, I drove past the big-box stores flanking LA's Sepulveda Boulevard and turned into the parking lot of a giant glass cube of an office building. It was one of those nondescript human hives, found in the suburbs of most American cities, where assorted professionals drone away from nine to five: transportation lawyers, loan processors, architects, orthodontists, and—most relevant to me that afternoon—psychiatrists.

I knocked on a door, and a late-middle-aged doctor with the central-casting trimmed gray beard invited me in. His wood-paneled office was decorated with aviation memorabilia—model planes, a vintage helmet, flags, pins. (Of all the shrinks' offices in all the towns in all the world.) He was an amateur pilot, it turned out. And, as I could have guessed from the moment I walked in, he was keenly interested in what my sister calls our family's "trail of tragedy." Chiefly my father's death in that plane crash in 1990, the near-loss of my mother to cancer when I was eight, her loss of her first son (my brother) to Down syndrome, but also my own close calls in various conflict zones. We talked for about an hour.

But it wasn't therapy I was after. The trials of juggling a career, a marriage, a growing family, an ailing mother, a financial betrayal by someone close to me, and my constant panic attacks had become more than I could bear. I sought salvation from the one source that had most reliably offered me comfort in the past: pharmacology.

Back in 2003, when I was a twenty-five-year-old print reporter, I had spent nearly six weeks in Iraq in the days after the US invasion. Nothing particularly bad had happened to me there. A colleague and I had done multiple reporting trips to Fallujah, an increasingly restive town that would soon become a byword for the insurgency, to report on the first attacks on US troops there. In the holy Shiite city of Najaf I had been swept away by a jubilant mob welcoming home an exiled cleric and was pinned against the doors of the mosque there until custodians opened them. Scary, for sure, but not something I considered traumatic at the time. Unlike some colleagues, I hadn't been shot at or detained by thugs (that would happen years later).

In fact, during the orgy of looting in those first few weeks after the US invasion, I witnessed what seemed the opposite of trauma: rapture. On several occasions Shiite men in the slums of Sadr City accosted me in the street only to wrap their arms around me. I stood there in shock as one man brought me in for a bear hug and cried out, "I love you, America! I love you, George Bush." When I asked him why, he spun around, lifted his shirt, and revealed the railroad yard of scars on his back and legs, the result of whippings in the regime's jails. Saddam's torturers favored electrical cables. And now Saddam and his henchmen were gone. Within a couple of months, almost no one was saying, "I love you, America."

For whatever reason, by the time I got back to my apartment in Tel Aviv, I had fallen into a funk—rarely leaving the apartment and watching *Black Hawk Down* on repeat. I was referred to a kindly Israeli psychiatrist who diagnosed me with mild depression and ADHD. He said my depression could easily be treated with a popular antidepressant called Paxil.

The first couple of days my mood and productivity sky-rocketed (perhaps the placebo hit me before the chemicals). I reached a near-manic state, driving my tiny Fiat Punto into the West Bank for all-night reporting stints. Within days the high leveled off. I wound up staying on Paxil, with a few hiatuses, for much of the next eighteen years.

In the meantime, my career was beginning its ascent. Jour-nalists typically want their stories heard or read by the larg-est, most influential audience possible. My own dream had been to be a swashbuckling Middle East correspondent for *The New York Times* or *The Washington Post* like Thomas L. Friedman and Anthony Shadid. I loved my job as a print reporter for *The Jerusalem Post*, whose editors offered me a long leash to report on almost any topic I wanted. But when I got the opportunity in 2005 to begin working with ABC News Radio, I jumped at it. The gig would be as a Jerusalem-based freelancer. ABC Radio broadcast short, fast-paced bul-letins at the top and bottom of every hour. My reports, which I would often deliver live, would typically last anywhere from twenty to thirty-five seconds. Since it was radio, I could read from a script either in the field or from a studio in Jerusalem.

ABC had sent me a CD of sample reports from its correspondents—an elite crew of virtuosos with godlike voices and always-perfect deliveries. As I began my own career in radio, I found myself prone to bouts of "nerves"—echoes of the full-fledged panic I had experienced that first time five years earlier as a Williams undergrad, though I was still so ignorant and ashamed of my panic that I never fully connected the experiences. It was "nerves" that would cause words to magically disappear from the pages I held firmly in my hands. It was "nerves" that caused my voice to crack or croak.

It rattled me: How could something that seemed so easy—just reading a short passage that I'd written myself—cause such sweating, breathless, word-mangling torment? I found I enjoyed the reporting work—gathering information, talking to people, writing up scripts—much more than the performative work.

A couple of years later I accepted a promotion as the Miami correspondent for ABC Radio. My wife, our two-month-old, Libby, and I packed up for South Florida. The staff gig came with a better salary, more responsibility, and something intensely coveted in the freelance world: a proper @abc.com email. I was now an official member of an elite tribe whose lineage of chiefs includes David Brinkley, Barbara Walters, and Peter Jennings. But that first year in Miami, whenever a big news story would break, my boss would burst into my radio booth vibrating with enthusiasm. He would ask, almost rhetorically: "You psyched about getting on air?!" It's been said that TV and radio reporters "live for airtime." So he was likely confused by my standard reply, a halfhearted, hesitant "Yeah . . ."

In April 2010, ABC Radio dispatched me to cover the BP oil spill befouling the Gulf of Mexico. All but moving into Louisiana's marshlands, I made friends with shrimpers, coast guard officials, and sources at BP, resulting in reporting and insight that gained notice. On a swampy Tuesday afternoon, in a moment that seemed pulled from a cheesy Hallmark movie about an aspiring TV journalist, I got "the call." It was the TV news desk—not the radio desk—asking if I would be willing to file a report on Diane Sawyer's *World News Tonight.*

"Um . . ."—deep breath—"yes."

Sawyer had apparently watched me on a weekend news show—I'd begun filing TV stories from the Gulf on the weekends with David Muir—and she liked my work enough that, two days later, she asked for me not just to appear on but to lead off her show. I had about two hours to write a script (which for a radio reporter was actually tons of time) before presenting the piece live.

In the space of less than a week, my career metamorphosed from that of a radio journalist in a satellite bureau to a mainstay of ABC's flagship newscast. I was now, in the words of *The Daily Beast,* one of Sawyer's "hunks," "the brow-furrowing newcomer who came up through ABC Radio but has a torso for TV." The sudden attention from the press, talent agents, and strangers on Facebook spawned ribbing from my colleagues and camera crews, who coined the nickname "the gunk hunk."

The live portions of my TV reports were actually shorter than my radio hits. But now I would be presenting not in some undisclosed radio booth but before a high-definition camera, consumed by an audience that had instantly grown by an order of magnitude. TV meant broader influence and a bigger salary. My "nerves" grew alongside them.

It was exactly what I had wanted, and precisely what I had feared.

The most obvious remedy to my "nerves," albeit a temporary one, was a flawless performance. Those came from time to time, wrapped in delicious dopamine that left me craving more. I found I was at my best when a shot involved a measure of choreography between camera, reporter, and control room—when it required a prop, or walking viewers through a tableau of destruction, or wading through oily water. That choreography helped take my mind off the precision of phrasing that I demanded of myself—and doing anything incorporating physical movement also seemed more authentically *me*.

During those first few months, when every live shot seemed like it could make or break a fledgling career, going on air felt like climbing into a boxing ring with the knowledge that a physical battering lay ahead. I would sometimes—fully aware of the cheesiness—psych myself up by humming the chorus to Eminem's "Lose Yourself": "You only get one shot, do not miss your chance to blow / This opportunity comes once in a lifetime."[*]

Perversely, the hair-on-fire nerves made my live performances appear more kinetic, earning me the reputation of someone who *thrived* on live TV. My efforts to ward off panic were interpreted by a *Good Morning America* executive producer as "energy" that "really punched through" to the audience. That got into my head, only ratcheting up the pressure.

Over the next few years, I almost never turned down an assignment, and my managers rewarded me by sending me everywhere—which of course meant more live reports. I most dreaded what should have been the "easy" live shots—just standing in front of a camera and offering a single thought in a couple of sentences. Their brevity came with an expectation of flawlessness, which meant that "ums," "uhs," repeated words, or brain farts were to be avoided. And anyway, how can anyone screw up fifteen seconds of talking? In those situations, I would have to physically hold myself together so

---

[*] The song is arguably the best-known ode to overcoming stage fright and panic, but lyrics from another song on that same album, "8 Mile," are probably just as appropriate: "Somethin' ain't right, hit the brake lights / Case of the stage fright, drawin' a blank like / Da-duh-duh-da-da."

tightly, spine so erect, that I'd walk away from the camera with Frankenstein stiffness, my lower back aching and my waistband dampened by the sweat coursing down my spine. It seemed to me that success in this industry depended on conjuring up a daily mirage and sustaining it for years. And I was certain that the next live shot would be the one in which my act was revealed to be an illusion—*I am not the person you see on your screen.*

You might now be thinking: If this job makes him so miserable, why the hell does he do it? It's a valid question. Like most jobs, mine can often be mundane. But sometimes we are witnesses to history. And, at its best, TV journalism reaches through the TV and grabs viewers by the lapels. In late February 2022, my producer Robert Zepeda and I crossed into Ukraine the day after Russia's invasion. We were among the first to report from the Krakovets crossing between Poland and Ukraine, where tens of thousands of refugees on the Ukrainian side were pressed up against the border gate, begging to be let through. Behind them was a twenty-mile-long traffic jam snaking back from the border. Many had run out of gas, abandoning their cars and lugging bags and children over gravel and slush to the border. These people would become the spearhead of the largest refugee crisis in Europe since World War II.

Men of fighting age were prohibited from leaving the country. We saw husbands and fathers bury their faces in the necks of their spouses and children, banking their scent before walking away to war, unsure if they'd ever see their loved ones again. Some never did. Mothers and children and fathers cried. As did we, along with so many viewers who tuned in to those broadcasts—bearing witness alongside us.

Later the same year in a series of trips, producer Angus

Hines and I reported on the emerging famine in East Africa, caused in part by soaring food and fuel prices, an indirect consequence of the war in Ukraine. In Kenya we met children who walked twenty-one miles every day to pick palm fruit, which has the consistency of shoe leather. They explained their goats had died and palm fruit was the only food they had eaten for weeks. In Somalian camps for the internally displaced, we interviewed mothers who had fled al-Qaida-controlled towns only to face losing their toddlers to malnutrition in a displaced-persons camp. Millions were in peril, and hundreds of thousands faced death, most of them children. Many Americans had heard little to nothing about the emerging famine so far away. Teleporting American viewers into a place they'd never go remains one of the great privileges of our work as journalists.[*]

It's not all selflessness, of course. I admit that I live for the adrenaline-infused you-can't-make-this-shit-up craziness that occasionally happens in the field. Take the 2016 capture of the narco kingpin Joaquín Guzmán Loera. You might know him as El Chapo, the Houdini-like drug lord who over the years broke out of *two* Mexican maximum-security prisons. He was on the lam again when one early January morning our news desk in New York heard rumblings of urban warfare in a small city of Los Mochis in Sinaloa, Mexico. There were reports of .50-caliber machine-gun fire, explosions, and a series of carjackings. We soon learned it stemmed from a nearly botched operation to capture El Chapo, who had squirted into the town's sewer system and nearly escaped again before being detained. Capturing the public's imagina-

---

[*] Our Somalia report for *World News Tonight* helped raise about $750,000 for hunger relief.

tion was a grainy bit of video posted on social media in which a gunman popped out from that town's sewer system, carjacked a vehicle, and sped off. Had that been El Chapo?

Later, when we landed in Los Mochis to cover the story, my producer Brandon Baur and I decided to head to the intersection at which the gunman had been filmed. We pulled over and tried to triangulate where the man might have emerged from. I started asking locals, and one man pointed to the center of the four-lane intersection. Our cameraman Mauricio and I scampered across the road looking for the manhole. With Baur blocking traffic and the camera rolling, I kneeled down and wedged my finger into a notch in the manhole cover. Pulling it up, I peered down and then muttered under my breath: "Holy fucking shit."*

Right there, leaning up against the sewer wall, was an M4 assault rifle with a grenade launcher. We had found El Chapo's escape route. Apparently, no one else had discovered it, including the Mexican military. The sewer wasn't very deep, less than five feet down. We ducked into the hole, careful not to disturb the weapon and trying to avoid turds and critters. I crab-walked, on camera, down the sewer, showing how El Chapo and his bodyguard must have escaped from their safe house a half mile away, then hopped out and carjacked their way to almost safety. Later, the Mexican military let us film his safe house and the trapdoor in a closet leading to a tunnel that opened up to that same sewer.

That bit of storytelling was not likely to win us an Emmy. But it was what we call in our industry "a TV moment," a string of nearly unforgettable images. It was the kind of thing that could simply not be captured (or even believed) in print

---

* That part was bleeped out.

or on radio. You had to *see* it unfold. Only the visual medium can do justice to moments like that.

The flip side of TV's validation, however, is a feeling of instant and constant judgment. Where a good segment might leave you feeling satisfied and elated, a subpar performance left you stoop-shouldered and deflated.

Too often I was in that latter camp. I suffered from textbook "imposter syndrome," a psychological phenomenon that disproportionately affects high-achieving people (particularly women and people of color) who are incapable of accepting or internalizing their success. Achievement can only be the result of the fraud we are perpetrating on everyone else.

It took years for me to understand that the "nerves" that long afflicted me were what you and I could now so plainly diagnose as panic attacks. My panics seemed to adhere to some lost law of physics: Panic cannot be created or destroyed. It is as constant and immutable as the speed of light.

During my years as a newspaper reporter, I developed a super-sloppy shorthand to prevent interviewees from peeking over at the (sometimes unflattering) descriptions I had written in my notepad. In later years, I had become so accustomed to secrecy about my panic that I applied that same indecipherable shorthand whenever I journaled about panic. In the service of self-denial, I prevented myself from easily peeking into my *own* thoughts. When I recently returned to those journal entries, I found time capsules of shame, filled with barely decipherable hieroglyphics.

SLEIGHT OF HAND

Hiding your vulnerability from others requires greater sleight of hand than hiding your own journal entries from yourself. I assumed that if people learned of my panic, I'd be seen as deadweight that the network would try to cut loose. To avoid that, I developed an ever evolving routine, part superstition, part hocus-pocus.

In my earlier years, when nailing each live shot felt essential to sustaining my near-accidental career in TV, I would fake napping in order to meditate for a few minutes—sneaking in a session in a parked car, or even while an unwitting producer was driving us to a live shot. Back then, it seemed even "needing" to meditate betrayed a kind of vulnerability I should avoid.

Twenty years earlier, my parents had dragged my chubby twelve-year-old self to a cheerless basement in Madison, New Jersey. Other parents sent their kids to sleepaway camp or schlepped them to piano lessons. But my post-hippie parents thought I could use a weeklong course in Maharishi Ayurveda's transcendental meditation. And so in August 1990 I ceremoniously received "my" mantra* and was taught the art of "gentle effortlessness," a skill requiring herculean effort: one must repeat one's mantra over and over without actually saying it aloud, or even hearing it in your head at any regular cadence or rhythm. Though later grateful for the gift of meditation, at the time I would have preferred watching mindless television and slurping Chef Boyardee, or even doing homework, to being indoctrinated into the "collective unconscious."

My other remedies weren't always so wholesome. In my years as a print reporter in the early 2000s, lots of journalists

---

* The maharishi make a big ceremony of bestowing upon their newly meditating clients what they tell you is an utterly unique mantra. They swear their inductees to an oath of secrecy. I solemnly kept that secret for decades until a friend bet me he had the same mantra. Turned out he did! It was "enga." Mantras are conferred by instructors based on age and gender.

still smoked, and many who "didn't smoke" bummed a cigarette here or there. Offering a cigarette, even if declined, was
an easy conversation starter with a potential interview subject. In the developing world, a smoke, or better yet a pack,
was a surefire way to make allies—especially among bored
and trigger-happy soldiers or police. Smoking seemed to mol-
lify my perpetual fidgetiness.

It also seemed to enhance some experiences—like breakfast with actor and lifelong smoker Sean Penn, who materialized at our out-of-the-way hotel in Baghdad in 2003. "Holy
shit, what's Sean Penn doing in Iraq?" He was sitting alone,
so my two reporting companions and I joined him at his table,
where we drank sludgy Arabic coffee, swapped stories for
hours, and of course smoked.

I have never suffered nicotine withdrawal, which made
quitting easy—and picking it right back up again just as easy.
There was the mild high of that first cigarette in a few months
or a year, and something soothingly familiar about the ritual
of snapping one of the perfect white sticks from a pack and
nimbly popping it in my mouth. Yet with each inhalation I
would mercilessly berate myself. *You stupid fuck. What are
you doing? You take such good care of yourself . . . Okay, I'll
let myself have one more smoke . . . Ahh, why are you so stupid?!* That feeling would be amplified when a colleague would
catch me smoking during one of my "off the wagon" periods,
prompting a shocked, "*You* smoke?"

Over the years I concocted superstitions around smoking, such as the notion that doing something so destructive
to my body might imbue it with supernatural protection from
anxiety.*

---

* Turns out shamans of the Shipibo tribe in Peru consider tobacco a sacred
plant and smoke pure tobacco incessantly during ceremonies. They believe the

The thing is, smoking makes you thirsty. It is also a diuretic, making you need to pee more frequently. Coffee, which I guzzle (half-caf or decaf these days), is a timeless companion to smoking and also a diuretic. Both make your mouth dry. Add a spoonful of anxiety, which can increase the urge to drink water, and you have a perfect pee storm on your hands.

Unsurprisingly, I constantly needed to go. TV journalists spend an unhealthy amount of time in cars, sometimes driving for hours from a hotel to the location of a train wreck/fire/tornado/shooting and then back again. On those long drives, I often required frequent pit stops, or if I was running late (and driving alone), I did what truckers do: pissed in a bottle. Rest assured, unlike some truckers, I have never hurled a so-called "trucker bomb" out the window.

I had other hacks aimed at reducing panic. Typically the control room in New York prefers that correspondents appear in front of the camera thirty minutes before a live shot. But prepositioning yourself means you are then being watched or at least monitored in the control room. This feels like what in the NFL they call "icing the kicker," when an opposing team makes a placekicker wait for as long as possible before a make-or-break field goal. The rationale is that the longer the kicker waits, the more time there is to think about the stakes involved, and the higher the chances of a shanked kick. So to avoid shanking a live shot, I would show up on the later side of "on time"—sometimes cutting it so close that the crew and control room may have suffered panic attacks themselves. (I am sorry, my friends.)

---

plant has properties that attract positive energies and ward off evil. As I noted earlier, they use a different species of tobacco, called *mapacho*, that is unprocessed and said to be not nearly as violently destructive as commonly sold cigarettes. By the way, they eschew alcohol, saying the spirit steals your soul.

In the beginning of my TV career, in the days of the Gulf oil spill, I did push-ups before airtime; people surely thought I was just a meathead. I wasn't sure why I did it, but it seemed to calm my nerves and keep me warm on chilly predawn mornings. Years later, after learning that mild exercise can reduce anxiety, I switched to jumping jacks or side twists—making a show of stretching a stiff back or warding off the early morning chill when in truth I was primarily trying to ward off panic. Alternatively, in the spirit of "fake it until you make it," I sought refuge in bonhomie, chitchatting with the photographer or the producer right up to the very last moment.

Sometimes it worked. Often, my tricks failed me. The resulting panic would invariably be followed by the familiar shame hangover: *Again? Another one? Why are you so damn broken?!*

The next car in this train of thought would be packed with worry. *Did I just conjure up a streak of chokes? Will I be the Joe DiMaggio of flubs? Can I ever do this job without thinking I'm going to die on air?*

IF YOU CAN'T BEAT IT, DRUG IT

By 2016, I needed more than mindfulness, cigarettes, and camaraderie. We had just moved from Miami to LA, where ABC has its West Coast bureau. It was wonderful to live so near to my in-laws, and particularly my mother-in-law, who insisted that cleaning was her therapy. Each time she came over, she would swap her street clothes for her superhero uniform of a patterned orange muumuu and rubber gloves and start scrubbing our kitchen.

The painful drawback of the move was the early wake-ups. *Good Morning America* airs at 7:00 a.m. Eastern time, which is 4:00 a.m. Pacific. This means that on too many mornings my alarm rings between 12:30 and 2:30 a.m., depending on where our team is located, our time slot in the show, and how far we need to travel to reach our live shot. My sleep schedule became a disaster, the panics had started to cluster, and my overall mood took a nosedive.

After a short hiatus, I wanted—no, I *needed*—to get back on antidepressants. And now that we'd moved to LA, I needed to find a new prescriber. All of which is why I found myself in that wood-paneled shrink's office with the all-too-on-the-nose model airplanes. I was no stranger to such offices. There was that first psychologist in middle school after my father was killed; then in high school it was a sweet former hippie. In college I had two, one motherly and gentle, followed by a stern Freudian. There was an ex-rocker therapist in Tel Aviv, and then the elderly psychiatrist who first prescribed me Paxil. When we moved from Jerusalem to Miami, someone set me up with an Argentinian therapist.

Regardless of the shrink, the geography, or the particular discipline they favored, we seemed to talk about the same stuff—over and over. So much discussion of family and trauma, pain and longing. Panic, however, never came up—because I didn't even know how to bring it up. It's one of the inherent problems with talk therapy.* A patient can "play" a therapist for years. It's possible neither of them will know it's happening.

This new psychiatrist I'd sought out in LA was different. He specialized in anxiety disorders and was a renowned expert in chemical dependency and opiate treatment. He became the first mental health professional I ever confided in about my panic attacks. It came almost as an aside.

He and I were on the same page. I had spent years talk-

---

* To be fair, it can be great for the treatment of specific issues at specific times.

ing to psychologists about my childhood, my attraction to risk, the struggle to balance family and career. If the level of my panic was any indication, talking alone wasn't enough to resolve the underlying issues. I needed to bring in the big guns. We both believed that some drug was the cure. We just had to find the right one, or the right combination.

By then I had been off antidepressants for about a year—like many patients hoping that they no longer need their medication. My new doctor agreed that Paxil was probably still worthwhile, given the overall benefits and lack of side effects I'd experienced on it previously. Plus, he said, studies had shown it had the ancillary benefit of reducing the incidence of panic. Why that was, no one was quite sure, and considering that many of my early panic attacks took place while on a steady diet of the stuff, it was clearly no panacea. But I was eager to give it another try. The knowledge that it might prevent *worse* panics could allow it to serve as a placebo.

Over the next couple of years, Paxil did curb my generalized anxiety, but it never seemed to put a dent in my panic attacks.

The doctor suggested Klonopin, a drug in the class of benzodiazepines, commonly prescribed to treat panic attacks. I had taken it once before. My team was in Mexico, having wrapped a shoot about surviving on a desert island. The shoot required me to jump from a helicopter about thirty feet into the shark-infested waters off Isla Tiburón in the Gulf of California. Under the guidance of survivalists, I then swam to shore, learning the skills to endure the next twenty-four hours or longer without food or water or shelter. When it was over, I was exhausted. Unfortunately we had booked a red-eye flight home to Miami, so my producer offered me a Klonopin to ensure I slept. I inadvisably washed it down with a glass of red wine. I woke up early the next morning in Miami, mildly groggy but happy to have slept the whole flight.

But I had not actually slept the entire flight. Our flight from Mexico City to Miami wasn't direct. The plane had stopped in Houston, during which time I had gathered my possessions, disembarked, walked to another terminal, and boarded another plane. I'd had conversations with colleagues and flight attendants. And yet I remembered none of it. Not a single memory. Suffice it to say, I thought it wise to avoid Klonopin.

Alternatively, the psychiatrist suggested Xanax, pre-scribed to manage all sorts of conditions under the broad banner of anxiety. My first experience with the drug, as a bereft twelve-year-old, certified its status as lifesaver during periods in extremis. The pill's familiar sweet bitterness was like the embrace of an old friend. It soothes us neurotics, smoothing out spikes of worry. It was so good at beating down the excessive rumination and circular thoughts that sometimes kept me awake, gently laying me down to rest. What was not to love?

I began carrying Xanax in a special compartment of my work bag as a "break glass" measure. Because Xanax begins having an effect within fifteen or twenty minutes, my doctor suggested I pop a pill shortly before a live shot. The problem was, we field reporters work in close proximity to producers and camera operators—often driving around all day in the same car. And "shortly before the live shot" is the most intense part of it, when we're usually scrambling and all together. I wasn't keen on anyone thinking I needed benzos to perform.

To keep up my overall facade of good cheer (which comes naturally) and imperturbability (not as much), I developed ways of smuggling a Xanax into my mouth. It would begin with an ostentatious rummaging in my backpack, as if to broadcast, *Just digging around clumsily here; nothing to see, folks*. I'd then quietly unzip the pocket at the top of my bag. Without taking the pill bottle out of the bag, I'd stealthily twist off the cap and select a pill, and slip it into my hand. By faking a cough or two, I could flick the pill into my mouth and swallow it dry. I'd like to think the Kabuki worked, though it increased both my anxiety and my shame. (Upon reflection, it's doubtful anyone would have cared if I had just taken out the bottle and swallowed a pill in full view.)

The starter therapeutic dose for Xanax (the generic version is called alprazolam) is .25 to .5 milligrams three times a day. I was taking single doses of .25 milligrams or .375 milligrams, which the doctor thought might suffice, if only as a placebo.* But neither the dosage nor the placebo was working. When I experimented and took enough to feel confident that panic could be averted—around .5 milligrams—it left me lethargic and not entirely *un*panicked. After a couple of years of sporadic use, I stopped. I didn't mind the notion of taking drugs to treat my panic. I did mind the sensation of *feeling* drugged while taking them and the constant uncertainty about whether they would work.

One day in 2017, I made a big ceremony of confiding in my agent that I suffered panic on air. His response: "You and lots of other people!" I was shocked. I had known that Dan Harris, my friend and colleague at ABC News, had had a major panic attack. His book *10% Happier* chronicles his evolution from a partier who seemed lost in the world to a person who found meaning in meditation. But "*lots* of other people"? My agent recommended I try propranolol, a pill long favored by TV personalities and performers the world over. Even profes-

---

* Many patients diagnosed with generalized anxiety disorder are prescribed as much as 4 milligrams per day. Dependence on benzos is pervasive. My doctor and I eagerly wanted to avoid that.

sional concert musicians find it particularly useful because it helps steady hands and fingers that might otherwise tremble while playing the piccolo or piano.

My doctor agreed that propranolol was worth a shot. And it did indeed prevent my heart from racing (and hands from shaking). But it didn't seem to slow the galloping thoughts before, and the brain fog during, a live report. That's because it blocks the effects of adrenaline but not anxiety. It, too, left me feeling lethargic afterward. I wound up using it only a handful of times.

Undeterred, my shrink and I continued to forage for the right drug in the great forest of pharmacology. He prescribed gabapentin, of a class of anticonvulsant medications meant to treat seizures by reducing "abnormal" excitement in the brain. It's often prescribed off-label for treatment-resistant mood and anxiety disorders and, increasingly, for PTSD. Side effects often include drowsiness and dizziness. I tried gaba a few times but recoiled at taking enough of it during the day to feel something.

Maybe the problem wasn't just my innate anxiety. Maybe it was ADHD? I had lugged that ADHD diagnosis around for even longer than the panic attacks. My LA psychiatrist gamely suggested Strattera, a nonstimulant drug approved by the FDA to treat ADHD. Much like many antidepressants, it takes weeks to take effect in your system. In those weeks, I suffered debilitating insomnia and an equally debilitating inability to properly digest food. After three months of sleep deprivation and diarrhea, the doctor and I decided to call it quits on Strattera.

Later I would try Adderall. But because I grew up before the Ritalin craze had fully caught on, taking it daily as an adult, with the rush it yielded, it was hard to shake the stigma that this wasn't a medicine that happened to be a stimulant; it was speed. Looking at the label after picking up my first pill bottle from the pharmacy didn't help: the generic name for Adderall is amphetamine salts. And while it helped me focus, it seemed to have little or no impact on panic. (Some psychiatrists later expressed surprise that I'd been prescribed a stimulant at all, since they're known to *increase* anxiety.)

My panic seemed powerfully resistant to any drug I was willing to take. We had tried mightily, but I was coming to terms with the plain fact: there was no magic pill. I would later learn this is not because of my body's failure to react properly to these medications. It's because, as we've seen, no one quite knows how the hell they work. According to Anne Harrington in *Mind Fixers: Psychiatry's Troubled Search for the Biology of Mental Illness,* most of the antidepressant drugs and benzos currently on the market were originally developed decades ago, and little new research has been done on drug development since the early 1990s. So, she writes, drug companies "responded to the lack of new scientific ideas about drug development by brilliantly marketing old drugs for new purposes."

I recently asked a senior official at a big pharma lobbying consultancy about this. I was hoping to report on work being conducted somewhere that would ease the pain of millions of my fellow panic and anxiety sufferers. I imagined they would take me to a lab where potential remedies for panic were being cooked up in giant vats. There had to be big money there, I figured.

The actual response: There may or may not be such studies in the works, and if there were, the person I spoke to wouldn't, for proprietary reasons, tell me anything about them. Thanks, big pharma.

Meanwhile, for all the struggle it entailed, my job continued to give me a sense of purpose (and, as important, a paycheck). I worked extraordinarily hard; I was dedicated to giving a voice to the voiceless. I also began to realize that I did not *want* to rely on a magic pill. I wanted to "be well." I was left fantasizing about completing a single live shot, just once, completely free of fear. When that seemed unrealistic, I fantasized even more often about quitting television entirely. My wife and I talked about it from time to time. She said she would gladly accept a reduced standard of living for our household if it meant her husband was less miserable.

THE LAST JENGA PIECE

Because I knew. I knew that, one day, a panic attack would pull the lynchpin Jenga piece from the tottering tower I'd built and it would all come crashing down. It's why I physically winced when I saw the call coming in on Tuesday morning, January 28, two days after my mistake. It was my boss. On the phone with her was a small group of executives. They had made a decision: I would receive a monthlong suspension. My head drooped down to my chest as I accepted the punishment, again apologizing for my error.

Within twenty-four hours, news of the suspension leaked to the media. I crafted a statement that read: "We are in the business of holding people accountable. And I hold myself accountable for a terrible mistake, which I deeply regret. I want to personally apologize to the Bryant family for this wrenching loss and any additional anguish my report caused."

In twenty years as a journalist, never had my words been cast so broadly. Hundreds of publications around the world reported it. The enormity of my error ensured that almost immediately it picked up steam—and venom—on social media. It made for the worst kind of name-and-face recognition—the kind we reporters often reluctantly have to report on.

There was a lot of shame in those weeks. But there was also some relief. Finally, as I had always expected, the jig was up.

CHAPTER 3

The Good Panic

I t was mid-February 2020, a couple of weeks into my suspension. Online, thousands of bylines over a twenty-year career in journalism were now buried under a single genre of headline: *ABC News Suspends Reporter Matt Gutman over Inaccurate Statement* (that was from CNN). Variations of that headline from hundreds of media outlets turned up in any Google search of my name. The results ran dozens of pages deep. A friend in PR said it would likely require years' worth of new bylines for Google's algorithm to sift out that pile of headlines. I asked him what you call a situation like this. He fired off his answer in a one-word text message: "infamy."

And then there were the looks. Mostly glances of compassion or curiosity. Whatever their motivation, I was desperate to get away from them. Really far away. The year before, I had befriended a family in Fairbanks, Alaska—snug up against the Arctic Circle. They had been breeding and training sled dogs for two generations, famous for how tenderly they treated their animals and how long the dogs lived. I reached out to the family, figuring this was as good a time as any to maroon myself in Alaska. They graciously offered me a place to stay. My wife, Daphna, recognizing the depths I'd fallen into in the preceding weeks—and maybe eager for a respite from my moping around the house—generously encouraged me to take a week to go process everything.

Upon arrival, one of the trainers put me to work helping harness, feed, and shoe the dogs.* My main gig would be cleaning the areas around their doghouses—in other words, poop scoop detail. I was given a shovel and a metal dustpan. I quickly learned that there is nothing quite as satisfying as chipping away at a frozen puck of dog pee and the *plink* when it pops out of the ice. The dogs themselves were the best therapy, rewarding their new janitor with kisses at every stop.

After staying a few days, I bid a grateful goodbye to the family and the dogs. I had decided to spread the six-hour drive south to Anchorage airport over a day and a half. The route takes you across the salt-bleached George Parks Highway, an asphalt ribbon through snow-blown wilderness. It's punctuated by Denali, the highest peak in North America—one of my bucket list destinations.

After about two hours on the road, I pulled into Denali National Park and Preserve and consulted my trail app. It recommended Mt. Healy as a moderately difficult, lightly trafficked trail with an elevation gain of about 1,700 feet. The app didn't mention the warnings I later found on the National Park Service website: that there is no marked trail to the summit, that "it's one of the steepest trails at Denali," and that "people have died in falls on Mt. Healy."

Oblivious, I parked and started hustling uphill. With the sun peeking through the clouds and a temperature of 10 degrees Fahrenheit, it was balmy for Denali in February.

---

* You would be surprised to know how much effort goes into caring for huskies' paws, which are shockingly fragile. One has to be especially cautious to avoid stepping on them. Trainers spend hours massaging ointment onto them.

I started unzipping layers as I chugged up the trail, energized by the majesty of the mountain range and the endorphins flowing through me. A few hundred yards from the trailhead it was just me, clusters of white spruce, and an occasional rabbit skimming along the surface of the snow like Jesus on water.

I had sturdy boots, warm clothes, a couple of protein bars, and a water bottle. Otherwise I was blissfully unencumbered—this was, after all, just a three-hour hike. When the trail disappeared, I stamped around for a bit trying to find it, but it just ended. Since I could see what I thought was the summit through cracks in the cloud cover, I decided to bushwhack toward it, basically crab-walking up the several hundred feet in elevation until I reached the top. The summit rewarded me with a tableau out of a Jack London novel—an expanse of arcing rivers, spruce forests, and the alabaster steeples of snowy peaks.

Exploring the ridge, I found an indentation the size of a kiddie pool where a moose had bedded down the previous night, leaving tufts of brown fuzz. The sun was getting low, and it was too steep to go back the way I'd come. I figured I'd wind my way down the mountain as if descending a spiral staircase. Eventually I would have to intersect the trail.

Initially the snow was knee-deep, and I developed a way to roll/flop down, which minimized effort and maximized fun. I was nature-drunk—intoxicated by the air, the vistas, and the endorphins. I took gee-whiz videos to show the kids once I got home. But farther down into the creases of the mountain, the snow became hip-deep, and flopping no longer worked. My shit-eating grin faded. I waded on, blindly trying to find "shallower" snow. But it all just looked like . . . well, snow. Traversing one ravine, I sank into snow as deep as I was tall.

My kingdom for a sure footing. Whenever I dug or tried to vault over the snow, the powder immediately refilled every cavity. This was frozen quicksand. Huffing from the exertion, I sagged onto my back to pull out my snow-encrusted phone. I had no reception on this side of the hill. I was imprisoned in soft snow, with little water left and one remaining protein bar. I was sweating now, my long johns stuck to my skin. With arctic night descending, I thought, *Holy shit, I could end up a human popsicle. I could be one of the people I've done stories about.*

Suddenly I felt the telltale pounding of my pulse, the galloping of my heart, the bugging of my eyes. The acute stress response I knew so well was releasing a lovely dose of adrenaline into my body. Samuel Johnson had it right when he said, "When a man knows he is to be hanged . . . it concentrates his mind wonderfully."

To rein in my fear, I took in a series of slow deep breaths. The worst of it passed, and several breaths in, my mind drifted to those bunnies I'd been seeing as I thrashed in the snow. How do snowshoe hares seemingly glide over the snow like hovercrafts? Ah, they're *snowshoe* hares.

Okay, I need to increase my surface area! I thought.

A tactic for escape now forming, my stress response also seemingly helped orient my internal GPS. I was completely lost but somehow, innately, I felt I knew the direction of the trail that I'd last been on about two hours earlier from a different side of the mountain.

The next fifteen minutes were spent thrashing over to a nearby spruce, buried so deep that only its crown peeked out above the snow line. I heaved myself onto its high branches like a life raft, then got to work snapping off as many as I could, silently apologizing to the tree. I began stuffing them into my boots, pants, and jacket pockets. I held some in my fists. It seemed ridiculous even then, but I was trying my best to turn myself into a human snowshoe.

I began flopping and flapping atop the snow. Less than an hour later, like a shipwrecked sailor, I washed back onto the trail, bedraggled and heaving from fatigue. I recorded a selfie video of embarrassed explanation, gratitude, and love to my wife and children. It's the kind of video that seemed perfectly necessary in the moment but which a later viewing proved too frothily crazy for public consumption. I never shared it with my family.

Stinking like a pine-scented car freshener, I hiked back to my rental car. I had narrowly missed a very miserable night, an embarrassing rescue, or worse. I realized that, in this instance, fear had saved me. As I would learn in the coming months, fear wasn't the enemy. Fear could be salvation. It was about having the right kind of fear at the right time.

HYPERACTIVATION

Having survived my great Alaskan bungle, I was zinging with lifeblood. Still, I dreaded going back to LA, where my mistake felt as fresh as ever. Which is why, when I returned, I felt like a kind of outcast. I never told anyone I worked with about the role of panic in the whole debacle. Panic was still shameful to me. Plus, such an admission would feel like a cop-out, an excuse for shoddy work—or, worse, a plea for sympathy.

I couldn't sleep in those days. I was waking up at 3:00 a.m.—but not for any *GMA* appearance. I would replay what happened on January 26 over and over. Masochistically, I kept Google Alerts on, which notified me of the dozens of articles about my suspension. Almost all of them were reported fairly. I also read some of the many thousands of comments on social media. Those were less fair. Many called for my firing or, better yet, my permanent banishment from the news. Some thought a much worse punishment was due.

I was experiencing the kind of social rejection that had instilled terror in me for a decade—the fear that something would blow my cover, revealing me not as the confident reporter you could throw into a combat zone or a flash flood, but as a hack. I had started a plant-based diet weeks earlier because I had read that it would help me heal from a recent shoulder injury. Add some agita to the mix and I had lost enough weight that people started to ask my wife, sotto voce, if "Matt . . . has, um [looks around furtively], *cancer*?"

It wasn't cancer. Something similar had happened to me about three years earlier. Reporting from Venezuela in late October 2016, I had been detained for five days, first by the national police and then by the country's infamous secret police (known by their Spanish acronym, SEBIN). During our first night being questioned, one officer entered the room, casually tapping a truck's dipstick on the palm of his hand. Fixating on it, I wondered which end of us the dipstick would go, "up the ass or down the throat," and which would be less damaging. Throughout the experience we stuck to obvious truth, that we were not spies or saboteurs but accredited journalists just there to tell the story of the children withering away in the country's hospitals.

Thankfully that dipstick was never used and we weren't physically harmed, but there were other unpleasant episodes, including an uncomfortably long period of being handcuffed, the threat of indefinite imprisonment because "you are CIA," a high-speed chase in Caracas, and the persistent rash, which came home with me. I convinced my hosts that I was *not* CIA when describing my duties as then host of the children's show

Sea Rescue. Using pidgin Spanish and pantomime, I tried to explain the premise of the show. I did not know the Spanish term for "sea lion," so I barked like one instead while slapping my hands together in front of me. They all laughed. After that, no one thought I was a spy. After our team's release was arranged and I returned to LA, I felt isolated and hyperfocused on my experience, which I journaled about manically for a couple of weeks.

Now, here I was in 2020, again in a similar hyperactivated state—sleeping little, eating little, stewing in rumination. I tormented myself with questions: Why was it that I seemed to be more afraid of the prospect of social rejection than a physically life-ending experience?

Those mornings alone in the house were clarifying. A career that seemed to hold limitless potential paths was now reduced to a single choice. I had to either get to the bottom of my panic attacks—or find a new profession.

I knew I couldn't possibly be alone in this struggle. Lots of people suffered from anxiety. Surely others, like me, suffered panic attacks in secret. I spent hours in my little home office scouring PubMed for studies on panic attacks. I began reaching out beyond my little carrel, talking to psychiatrists and psychologists. They were amazingly sympathetic.

Many of the experts offered the same advice: Panic attacks are a trick played by our brains, not the terminal disease I had made them out to be. There was nothing fundamentally wrong with me. I simply had to learn to outtrick my mind. (As you'll soon see, this advice wasn't 100 percent on the mark. But it came from a good place.)

It was reassuring to know that I wasn't broken, but those panics didn't *feel* like tricks; they felt like a pile driver. I kept asking those psychologists the annoying question common to children and journalists: "But *why?*" Why do we humans, highly evolved species that we are, still suffer from maladies like mine. Why hasn't panic been selected out over thousands of generations? Gradually it drew me to broader questions: Why do we suffer anxiety and panic at all? Where did all this worry come from? And how could it possibly be useful to us?

Like so many parents, mine had always taught me not to "care what other people think of you." But what if the old adage, fruitlessly battered into our minds, had it all wrong?

DID DINOSAURS WORRY ABOUT ASTEROIDS?

Revisiting my *Mr. Bean Goes to Alaska* moment on Denali, it became clear to me that, in the right setting, the suite of symptoms I associate with panic could be seen not as the brain's kryptonite, but as its superpower.

Here's what we might see if we rewound the tape of my ill-fated hike to the moment I recognized the possibility of life-threatening peril: From center field in my brain, the amygdala jump-started my sympathetic nervous system. The nearly immediate result was the release of adrenaline, initiating my fight-or-flight response. This was the surge of fear I felt when I realized I could end up a human popsicle. When the threat persisted (I was still neck-deep in snow), my hypothalamus ordered the release of cortisol, which prolonged my body's state of readiness against danger, helped me brainstorm a solution, maintain stamina, and ultimately scrabble to safety.*

I wanted to understand why our systems worked this

---

* The hypothalamus is in charge of the four F's: fleeing, fighting, feeding, and fornicating. It's the hormone factor, directing glands in our body to secrete hormones such as adrenaline, cortisol, oxytocin, and vasopressin.

way at all, and why my body seemed to flip the panic switch even at moments when I wasn't in life-threatening peril. So I reached out to Stanford researcher Robert Sapolsky. Sapolsky specializes in biology, neurology, and neurological sciences, not to mention being a noted primatologist who spent decades studying the social behaviors of savannah baboons in Africa.* He offered me a SparkNotes version of the origins of fear.

Sapolsky estimates that adrenaline and cortisol have been around for about five hundred million years—fifty million years before the dinosaurs, way back when vertebrates were just taking our first wobbly steps on this hot planet. Dinosaurs themselves developed fairly complex brains; still, they were not, in Sapolsky's words, "sitting around saying, *Like, shit, what if an asteroid hits Earth?*"

That's because, evolutionarily speaking, fear is old and worry is new. Dinosaurs experienced fear; they were driven to flee or fight based on stress responses. Fear and stress only reflected the next thirty seconds of their lives, Sapolsky explained. The reptilian brain of a sauropod, noticing a T-rex's advance, mustered an acute stress response that sent it running. But assuming it successfully evaded its predator, the sauropod's brain lacked the capacity for the follow-up thoughts that we know as worry or anxiety. *Why did that T-rex target* me? *Maybe there are other T-rexes in the neighborhood? What if this is a trap? Did anyone see me almost get eaten? Will my herd think I'm a bad sauropod for almost getting eaten?* A sauropod couldn't be anxious in this way if it tried.

---

* But wait, there's more: when he and I spoke, in addition to juggling his work at Stanford and writing his own book, he was working on a musical theater production with his wife.

Along came the apes, roughly twenty to twenty-five million years ago. They boasted a remarkable innovation: they got scared sooner. Chemically, early apes (and current humans) do this by releasing glucocorticoids, a class of hormones that enable the body to make maximal use of adrenaline. Priming an animal to be a fraidy-cat earlier than absolutely necessary offered a huge evolutionary advantage. By recognizing threats in advance, an ape could muster a stress response earlier and thus move to a safer perch, farther from its predator, rather than waiting to be chased and running pell-mell for its life. It also allowed the ape to avoid ancillary risks of such a retreat, like being trampled or being hurt in a fall. This was a nifty evolutionary development; it enabled not just survival but *planning*.

Given evolution's tendency to never leave an adaptation well enough alone, the great apes (chimps, bonobos, orangutans, gorillas, and their ancestors) fine-tuned this innovation. Sapolsky estimates that around five to seven million years ago, at about the same time that the earliest hominins are believed to have branched off from the great apes, apes developed the capacity for *abstract* fear. Being chased by a lion was no longer required to trigger an acute stress response. Now just sensing a lion lounging on the far edge of a clearing in the savannah was enough to get baboons screaming out alarms and moving away.

It was a kind of biological insurance policy more valuable than any claw or fang: pay a little energy now and save a lot later. An ape could now expend, say, fifty calories getting anxious, moving elsewhere, and avoiding a lion (or a rival). That's better than expending hundreds of calories running for its life and possibly losing contact with its troop in the process. And it's a hell of a lot better than being eaten for lunch.* Turned out that being scared sooner really was hugely advantageous—adaptive, in the language of evolution.

Fast-forward a few million years and our genetic human ancestors had become worrying savants. Their ability to think about a time other than the present moment paved the way for many forms of planning: seasonal hunts, storing food, the creation of tools for future use.† As Sapolsky jokes, they began "doing gloriously on marshmallow tests," referring to the famed 1970s experiments that measured a child's ability to delay gratification. Worrying about the future helped lead to our gift for symbolism; early hominins no longer had to physically lay eyes on a predator or competitor to trigger an acute stress response. It was now enough just to see a painted image of a lion on a cave wall or listen to a story about a lion encounter around the campfire.

It was only in the last 20,000 years or so, Sapolsky says, that we truly honed the skill of abstraction. Today I can be standing in front of a conceptual piece at the Museum of Modern Art, allowing my brain to wander, when all of a sudden the idea of social judgment (my personal predator) will pop up in my mind, triggering the kind of acute stress our primate ancestors only felt when facing down a predator in the savannah.

It was probably at this point—maybe about a thousand generations ago, a blink of an eye in evolutionary terms—that our body's useful servant anxiety became its sometimes mas-

---

* In case you're wondering, the sum total caloric value of a human is estimated to be about 125,000 calories. We know that because a scientist spent a large part of his career studying cannibalism in Paleolithic societies, even breaking down the caloric value of each part of the body, like thighs and arms.

† Psychologist Judson Brewer, author of *Unwinding Anxiety: New Science Shows How to Break the Cycles of Worry and Fear to Heal Your Mind,* counters that worry is not necessary for planning and that anxiety is often an entirely useless habit, one we can train ourselves out of.

ter. We became so good at symbolism that, for some, the response to the mere possibility of a threat could be more damaging than the threat itself.

THE SQUIRRELY BABOON

Sapolsky has spent decades studying a single population of baboons in Kenya because, he says, "baboon societies are ironically a lot like Westernized humans. We're ecologically privileged enough that we can invent social and psychological stress. Baboons in the Serengeti, who only work three hours a day to meet their caloric needs, are similarly privileged."* And also like humans, observed Sapolsky, baboons end up spending a lot of their free time "being horrible assholes to one another," particularly the males, which engage in pitiless harassment solely for harassment's sake.

Sapolsky isn't sure whether baboons suffer panic attacks, but he says it's evident that many suffer from anxiety. He described a hypothetical scenario in which a baboon male has somehow snagged a gazelle (baboons are omnivores). It's the Serengeti on a midsummer's day. The sun is high overhead, driving baboon competitors into the relative cool of the shade of an acacia tree. The grass is tall, providing a screen of privacy—ideal for a solo snack of gazelle tartare. Our baboon is wrist-deep in gizzard when he stops eating and looks around. Is a predator coming? Is a higher-ranking baboon coming to steal his meal? Or maybe a male baboon is seen merely napping nearby, a seemingly inconsequential action except for the fact that the napping male is of higher

---

* Apparently, being a baboon is a pretty cushy gig. Many hunter-gatherer societies studied by scientists today, like the Hadza in Tanzania, spend twice the amount of time meeting their caloric needs.

rank—which would entitle him to pilfer our subject's hard-won meal.

The baboon's twitchiness—measured as the frequency with which he looks up from his meal to ensure he's not attacked or bullied—helps scientists like Sapolsky quantify the animal's anxiety. The more scanning of the horizon and the less eating, the more anxious the animal. For baboons, as with many social animals, it turns out that seeing threats where none exist is negatively correlated with rank—meaning, the lower the rank of a baboon, the higher his anxiety. It makes sense: lower-status baboons enjoy less access to food and females and make easy targets for baboon bullies. Yet there's a crazy twist: being a *higher*-ranking male means relatively low stress, but being the *highest*-ranking male—the CEO of a troop—comes with lots of stress and consequently poorer health. Those baboon bosses find themselves constantly looking over their shoulders and engaged in battles to retain their primacy.

In the short term, the adrenaline and cortisol released by the stress response help you get through jams. But for baboons, and for humans, chronic activation of cortisol during periods of stress can cause ailments, including digestive trouble, heart disease, high blood pressure, stroke, sleep problems, weight gain (from pumping so much glucose into your system), memory and concentration impairment, and depression.

It's a head-scratcher: How can anxiety be both a highly useful adaptation and so very unhealthy? The answer to this evolutionary paradox may be found, indirectly, in peacocks.

PEACOCKS ARE SEXY

For years, the man considered the father of evolutionary sciences harbored a particular hatred for peacocks. Charles

Darwin was so vexed by the apparent paradox of a peacock's decadent plumage that he reportedly grew disgusted by the mere sight of the flightless bird. Peacock plumage seemed to punch a hole in his theory of evolution—that successful replication of a species depends on a creature's "fitness," its ability to survive.

By that logic, wondered Darwin, how could a five-foot-long caboose of multicolored feathers—which screamed to predators, *Here I am, come and get me!,* and that made the animal slower to get away from its predators—be *useful* to a peacock's survival?

Darwin's elegant answer was that plumage does not, in fact, make a peacock "fitter." It does not make him stronger or hardier. It makes him sexier. Darwin eventually concluded that the only conceivable answer to the riddle was that "we must suppose [peahens] admire [the] peacock's tail, as much as we do." Peahens were attracted to peacocks with the biggest, brightest plumage.

This is said to be how Darwin managed to square the circle of "natural selection," which, when tweaked, became a theory scientists call sexual selection. The game of life was not just about the survival of the fittest. Darwin understood that individuals in a species survive by adapting traits that both make them robust *and* promote procreation. At some point in peacock evolution, more elaborate fans began to signal health and virility. Those were traits a peahen found attractive because it meant they would be passed on to the amorous couple's chicks.

Peacock plumage would seem to be what's known as a maladaptation. It's caused by a runaway process in which animals keep selecting for an adaptive trait until it becomes more harm than good. Peahens saw signs of health, or something else they really liked (no one has been able to ask them), in bigger and brighter plumage, giving peacocks with the right plumage a reproductive advantage. Fast-forward thousands of generations and this massive, kaleidoscopic train of feathers became too much of a good thing, encapsulating the trade-offs inherent in sexual selection: what's sexy may not always be healthy.

All of which brings us back to worrying. Scientists believe that runaway anxiety, which can beget anxiety disorders, is a similar maladaptation, a human version of a peacock plume. Across the millennia, evolution selected for bigger and smarter brains that allowed our ancestors to plan hunts more efficiently—not to mention paint, sing, and dance, but also to worry better.*

Evolutionary biologists say there's a reason our worry has persisted, despite its mostly harmful effects on our body. They point to something called a selective or genetic bottleneck. The bottleneck generally results from a massive crisis—an asteroid plunking into earth, a once-in-a-century contagion that kills off a sizable percentage of a population, or a cata-strophic drought. The very small percentage of a population that survived had a quality the others lacked. For gazelles, that could be a trait that enabled their kidneys to cope with a historic drought on the savannah. While in good times hyper-efficient kidneys lead to kidney stones or water retention that could slow their running, when that once-in-a-century drought comes, individual gazelles with those weird kidney issues can unwittingly become the key to a species' survival, passing on their super-efficient use of water to their fawns.

In primates and humans, Sapolsky posits, maybe anxiety

---

* Obesity is the result of another once-adaptive trait turned maladaptive. We evolved to super-efficiently store calories as fat, enabling many a primate or human to survive periods of famine. But that has left us ill-equipped to live in a world where the problem is not too little fat, but too much.

or undirected dread became a kind of secret sauce. Most of the time, life is boring and repetitive, and anxiety is a useless, even harmful, feature that makes the nebbishy ape a target of bullies. But every so often a cataclysm comes; equilibrium is punctuated. It could be a virus, an invasion from a neighboring tribe, a German man with a funny mustache. All at once, the nervous Nellies' annoying motto of "better safe than sorry" gives them a jump on the competition, ensuring their DNA lives on.

It's counterintuitive, Sapolsky acknowledges. "When you look at [evolutionary] blinks of half a century, having that genetic profile of anxiety is so damn maladaptive. For instance, major depression is on the average shortening life expectancy by ten years and anxiety disorders vastly increase your odds of cardiovascular disease." It's harmful enough, in fact, that Sapolsky postulates that if you were to go "away and come back 10,000 years from now, everyone should be a Zen monk, because selection has eliminated the mood-disorder neurotics from the gene pool." Meaning, the trait that afflicts so many millions of people *should* theoretically go the way of Neanderthal brows and primate tails—consigned to the oblivion of evolution.*

It hasn't yet and, Sapolsky says, likely won't for a long while.

It may be reassuring, on an evolutionary scale, that eventually we could grow out of anxiety. Unfortunately for us panickers, our lifetimes are lived entirely in those "evolutionary blinks." Our bodies continue to mount the same response to imagined threats as they would to a lion lunging toward us. I needed help now—not in a million years.

---

* Don't get too excited. Many other scientists and psychologists I've spoken to say this will never happen.

CHAPTER 4

A Thousand False Alarms

A couple of years ago I started following a guy on Instagram who calls himself Liver King. At the time, he had a couple hundred thousand followers, whom he calls "primals" and to whom he preached the "ancestral lifestyle."* That number has since grown into the millions. He is articulate, incredibly entertaining, and enviably unselfconscious. He never wears a shirt on camera—even in winter—and he calls his wife "Liver Queen" and his sons "Liver Boys." He perpetually stays in character—he likes to say that he killed his previous self, Brian Johnson, years ago and that only Liver King survives. He has tractor treads for abs and anchor chains for arms, the product of his "barbarian" workouts (and, he later admitted, steroids). He gets plenty of sleep and avoids smartphones (he has a social media team that does most of the posting). His post-workout breakfast has him loading up on the kind of fuel he needs to get "swole": a slab of raw liver, raw bull's testicles, four to six raw eggs, homemade yogurt, a

* Sleep, eat, move, shield (avoiding phones, plastics, and unhealthy crap), connect (basically walk barefoot on the earth), cold (plunges), sun, fight (hunt), and bond. Most of which are commendable goals that would likely make anyone's life better—though I'm not sure if the hunting is necessary.

concoction of duck fat, almond butter, gelatin, creatine, and bone marrow—also raw. He also really likes to eat the raw bull's testicles, which have the texture of ceviche, on camera.*

Ah, to be Paleolithic. The idea has come into vogue that before humans began to domesticate animals and grains, we spent our lives roaming a veritable Garden of Eden. We gorged on freshly hunted meat, nuts, and succulent, low-hanging, non-GMO fruit. We logged 20,000 steps a day while hauling mammoth parts around, giving us rippling eight-packs and glutes that could crack walnuts. The constant foraging and hunting meant we marinated in nature, offering our brains the daily Xanax of the outdoors as well as plenty of vitamin D. With new rocks to find and throw, new herds of mastodon or wild sheep to chase off cliffs or spear, new fungi to taste-test—*delicious or deadly?*—there was constant novelty. Forget the 1950s; these were the true good old days. Given the reportedly surging anxiety rates of humans in the developed world—and a particularly alarming spike in young people—it's easy to romanticize our cave-dwelling ancestors, who we might imagine lived simpler, richer, and more health-ful lives. Hence the appeal of someone like the Liver King and his supposedly neo-Paleolithic lifestyle.†

Archeological and ethnographic evidence disabuses us of the premise of so-called "manthropology"—the notion that paleo men were uniformly stronger, faster, healthier, and hap-

---

* Just as this book was being finalized, I spent a day with Liver King at his Texas ranch. Post-steroids, he has upped his testicle eating to every several hours.

† The Liver King also asserts that our ancestors didn't brush or floss their teeth and didn't get cavities because they nourished their teeth from the inside out, including through the consumption of liver and egg yolk, not to mention plenty of sunshine. There may be some truth in what he says, though science is pretty clear that broken and decayed teeth killed plenty of our ancestors and certainly caused much pain.

pier. For one thing, evidence shows us that early humans were substantially wirier than the beefy Liver King.* And most died young. The fossil record from the heyday of Paleolithic times—around 30,000 years ago—shows that most adults died before their thirtieth birthdays, and child mortality was off the charts. Their lives were often literally Hobbesian: nasty, brutish, and short. Broken bones were mended jankily, injuries lingered, and disease was often a death sentence—an infected splinter wound could kill you. That's to say nothing of many mental illnesses, like schizophrenia, which likely existed at similar rates to today. Though it may be hard to believe, multiple studies have found Paleolithic societies (up until about 12,000 years ago) to be way more violent than modern ones.

There were just so many more ways for humans to meet an untimely death back then. Consequently, there were so many things to fear.

For the sake of argument, let's lump all human fear into two very broad categories. In that first bucket let's put anything we might consider fear of physical harm—anything that could maim or kill one of our ancestors or their offspring. This includes starvation, falling rocks, drowning, disease, thirst, bears, lions, and those murderous assholes from the rival cave group across the valley.† This bucket of fear offers immediate and obvious routes toward death.

Now let's look at the second bucket. Into it let's put what we might call social fears. While the objects of these fears

---

* In December 2022, he made his bombshell steroid confession (though many in the fitness world had long suspected his use of steroids and human growth hormone), admitting he'd been using performance-enhancing drugs for about four years.
† To be clear, this is an oversimplistic rendering of human fears, which are many and varied.

offered a less direct path toward a painful demise, in the long term they could be just as deadly. This requires a little more explanation, but it's essential to breaking down our damaging misconceptions of anxiety and panic today. So bear with me.

WELCOME TO THE TRIBE

Evolutionary psychologists believe that emotions came long before language. For millions of years, primates and other mammals were warned of imminent threats by, for instance, the look of fear on their groupmates' faces or a distress call that loosely translated to "RUN AWAY!" *Homo sapiens* fine-tuned linguistic communication such that they could convey far more complex ideas: "Hey, Bork, look there. At far end of clearing, lion with scar over eye. That lion tried to eat Mok last moon." This kind of communication allowed humans to get a lot better at surviving than their predecessors, despite our relatively puny physical strength and equally sorry speed. (Usain Bolt is likely the fastest human to have lived, but his top speed is slower than an average hippo's.)

This is why, before the invention of the wheel or the dis-covery of fire, the most profitable human venture (in terms of calories earned, calories saved, and human DNA replicated) was arguably our brain's ability to transmit packets of detailed information to one another—that is, communication.*

The fine-tuning of fear over many hundreds of thousands of years, along with our eventual ability to pack tremendous amounts of information into a series of sounds, came with a suite of other mental innovations that blew the rest of the ani-

---

* Hominins were the only primate lineage that evolved language, because hominins were the only great apes that evolved as cooperative extractive for-agers, simultaneously adapting for enhanced capacities to coordinate and for enhanced capacities to physically manipulate their environment.

mal kingdom away. We got even better at planning. Humans became able to anticipate changing seasons, preparing warmer loincloths, drying and storing mastodon jerky. We were able to coordinate upcoming hunts, foraging missions, our seasonal moves down the glacier, even the next tribal dance in homage to our earth mother goddess. Forget Facebook: hunter-gatherer lives literally depended on the strength of their social networks.

Our group was our everything. If you're a zebra and get attacked by a lion, you're screwed. The rest of your herd is gone before your entrails have hit the ground. But if Mok were to be attacked by a lion with a scar over its eye, he could be reasonably assured that his human herd would scream like hell, hurl some rocks and spears, and try to chase off the predator, then try to nurse their comrade back to health. Our species thrived thanks to networks of humans cooperating—offering mutual protection and communal child-rearing. In fact, grandmothers, and their ability to care for their grandchildren, are arguably why human moms have been able to produce many more surviving offspring in their lifetime than ape moms. (It's also why I'm so grateful to my muumuu-wearing mother-in-law.)*

Cooperation extended beyond the home; it found us associating with humans who weren't kin. It's one thing to co-

---

* In fact, it's possible that if it weren't for *Homo sapiens'* compulsion for co-operation, you would likely be crawling around on all fours right now. Apes managed to develop a knack for walking on their knuckles, which enabled them to carry very small things in their curled fists. Not a bad trick. But humans took schlepping to another level. One leading theory for bipedalism posits that sharing food—first with our mates and then with a wider group—led to the emergence of walking on two legs. Try it: it's really hard to carry a dripping honeycomb or a hunk of animal carcass while on all fours. Walking upright allowed humans to haul things back to a central location—where fragile young ones and their mothers would be safer—rather than bring the more vulnerable in a group to the site of the kill.

operate with people with whom we share a child or who carry half, a quarter, or even the roughly 3 percent of DNA of our second cousins. It's another to closely cooperate with lots of non-relatives. Being able to harmoniously work with family and friends meant that we could expend around half as many calories fulfilling our caloric requirements as most apes did. Over time our bodies could shed calorie-consuming muscle and bone density; we no longer needed King Kongian physiques to survive.

But what happens when a human refuses or fails to cooperate with their group? If forming and maintaining social connections was a matter of life and death—as important as access to food and water—how did you ensure that everyone played their part, rather than simply freeloading off the group? Welcome to the world of paleo punishment, which often took the form of shame and rejection.

Let's go back to those buckets of big human fears. If the first was fear of death by lion, hailstorm, infected splinter, etc., the second contained what I call social fears. Boiled down, this second group represents our fear of *expulsion from the tribe*.

We might imagine what that looked like to our cave ancestors: Shirk your duty the first time and you might earn a dirty look from your tribe's elders. But be a serial shirker of your duties, then eat too many of those funny mushrooms and accidentally step on your group's sacred earth mother figurine, and you could be excommunicated from the group altogether.*

---

* Ethnographic evidence suggests that the most hated of all non-cooperators were bullies. Bullies, who show aggression solely for egocentric reasons, "threatened the fabric of cooperation through violence and the threat of violence," writes Kim Sterelny in her paper "Cooperation, Culture, and Conflict." Research shows that bullies were often dealt with in the harshest ways, including capital punishment.

Many mammals could survive expulsion or a solitary life. Not *Homo sapiens.* Remember, our tribe gave us security, sustenance, and safety, enabling us to survive long enough to make babies and even grandbabies. Expulsion meant roaming the savannah or the jungle alone, where the chances skyrocketed of being eaten by another animal, dying from starvation, or suffering a debilitating fall. Social rejection could, in other words, be a death sentence.

Paleo punishment may sound harsh, but it wasn't arbitrary. Yale professor of social and natural science Nicholas Christakis says early humans practiced punishment and ostracism not out of cruelty but because, in the right circumstances, this improved the welfare of the group at large. Shunning freeloaders or other individuals who diminished cooperative behavior (like bullies) made the group stronger. Enforcers could earn social brownie points, and the release of dopamine that came with it. The threat of shunning worked well, too. You either got with the program or got kicked out. *Listen, Zek, you saw that Bork was expelled from the cave last rain season—better stop playing with your rock collection and start skinning that mastodon.*

Furthermore, studies have shown that being highly sensitive to social cues (but not reactive when detecting them) is actually an adaptive advantage. This means that, even though being sensitive to others' moods and caring what others think can be painful, it can, on balance, be a very good thing.

You might be thinking: But I don't live in a cave and I am not a hunter-gatherer. *You* know that, but your body doesn't. Like it or not, tens of thousands of generations of this exact kind of fretting are stamped onto your genes. "We have this dramatic, innate, 60,000-year-old, super-deep response to social evaluation," says Mitch Prinstein, a professor of psychology and neuroscience at the University of North Carolina, the chief science officer at the American Psychological Association, and author of the book *Popular.* "We can't pretend that we don't care about popularity . . . We do care, it's happening to all of us, it's biological. This is what makes us human, our ability to hurt, and to have this instinct to be sensitive to our social environments. That's why we survived compared to the Neanderthals and other species."

Shunning was not only something that happened *to you;* it was something that happened *in you.* Multiple studies have determined that social rejection spikes our inflammatory response and depresses our immune system. It makes sense: If we are alone in the wild, inflammation increases protection against possible injury or animal attack. And since we are no longer around virus-shedding humans in our cozy cave, what's the point of wasting energy powering our immune system?

Another study demonstrated that avoiding rejection is so central to our human survival that our brains react to *social* rejection as if it were *physical* pain. The study had dozens of volunteers play a frisbee-like video game called *Cyberball* inside an fMRI machine as researchers monitored their brains' reactions. In the first round, participants were allowed to "join" a game of *Cyberball* in progress. Later they were given an arbitrary reason for being excluded from the game and were forced to watch as others played without them. That rejection lit up brain images in a region of the brain associated with physical pain. The bigger the social rejection, the bigger the ouch.

This helps explain why the fear of social rejection is at the heart of many of our most familiar woes today: our social anxiety, our fear of public speaking, our agoraphobia. Those manifestations of our fear of social rejection may have kept us alive.

And what better reminder of the dangers of social rejection and running afoul of your group than a panic attack? As anyone who has experienced panic attacks will tell you, they are not soon forgotten.

Randy Nesse, the evolutionary psychiatrist at Arizona State, says humans are primed for panic.* He believes our brains would prefer a thousand false alarms to a single missed social or sensory cue.† In our conversations, Nesse repeated a phrase that has resonated with me ever since: "This [panic] is perfectly normal."

It is hard to emphasize enough the relief those four words gave me. Nesse's message was that the blast of anxiety we panic sufferers face isn't a glitch in the system. It is part of our fundamental programming.

The stakes for social threats may not be as obvious or immediate as those for physical ones, but our primal fear of them is no less real. And it's not just expulsion or rejection; we fear losing whatever social status we've worked to gain. Moreover, we've evolved to the point that we've become sensitive to the barest hint of social rejection—from a minutely cocked eyebrow to the stirring of a frown.

Managing a few dozen relationships in a cave 40,000 years ago would have been taxing enough. Managing hundreds of relationships—not to mention the interplay of total strangers in a city or town, or on social media—is enough to bring

---

* Numerous studies show that humans are still primed to fear snakes and spiders, for instance, even though the vast majority of modern humans will never encounter a deadly one in their lifetimes. According to Nesse, that's because our DNA has been wired to remember threats that persisted for many thousands of generations of human existence.

† This is called "signal detection theory." The body has a similar philosophy of pulling the fire alarm when it comes to almost every possible danger, including vomiting, coughing, fever, and pain.

all but the most insensitive among us to the brink of social awareness overload.

THE NORMALS

All this talk of status, prestige, and social rejection got me thinking about groups. What exactly was *my* group? When standing before the camera delivering a live shot and trying not to have a public meltdown, exactly what status did I fear losing, and from whom?

Ahead of most ABC News live shots, the anchor will introduce the correspondent with their title. My title has been "Chief National Correspondent" since ABC offered it to me in early 2018. It seemed an honor, though not something I had asked for or felt I deserved. For years, every time an anchor uttered the words "Chief National Correspondent" as I was about to go on air, I would recoil.

Though I am very good at what I do, when I would watch our ABC News programs, I'd marvel at the smoothness of my colleagues' writing, delivery, or mastery in the field. The addition of that title reawakened my imposter syndrome. And imposter syndrome can be a self-fulfilling prophecy. The more certain you are that you don't deserve what you've earned, the more it weighs on you. For me, that meant added anxiety, only amplifying the risk of a panic attack, proving what the skeptic-in-chief (me) always suspected: I am not worthy.

On many nights of the week, David Muir's flagship half-hour news show, *World News Tonight,* will be the most-watched broadcast on television, with between eight and ten million viewers. A common question I get is: "Don't you get nervous thinking that millions of people are watching?" The honest answer is no. I am sure those millions of dedicated viewers are wonderful people. But psychologically speaking, they are not the ones I worry about.

The audience I fixate on is the small tribe sitting in that darkened cave of a control room in New York City, illuminated by a hearth of flickering monitors: the anchors, network executives, and producers of *World News Tonight* or *Good Morning America*. Only they matter because, just as in the cave groups of 40,000 years ago, they have the power to judge whether my reports have made the group stronger or weaker. If they assess that something I've done has weakened the group, they have the power to shun me—for failure, violating a taboo, or freeloading. (To be clear, this is not an actual depiction of how things work at ABC. It's just how it used to appear inside my mind. These people have only been supportive.)

Grasping the intricacies of our evolution as a species, which leaned so heavily on cooperation, helped me understand why each live shot mattered so much to me. Each time I went on air, whether I knew it or not, I was trying to prove myself worthy of membership in this illustrious tribe. Ninety-five percent of the time—even during some of my panics—I "punched through." The nerves might even have improved my performance. Still, doing so night after night exacted a psychological and physical toll.

I thought back to what Plutarch described as "sudden foolish frights." That seemed wrong to me now. For tens of thousands of generations, our collective experience has genetically reinforced in us the sense that social rejection is as threatening as any predator. It's why, as Randy Nesse observed, our bodies would rather blare out countless false alarms about the risk of social expulsion than risk missing a single real one—because the danger of being made an outcast is as real as any physical pain we might face.

Seen in that light, maybe our "frights" aren't so "foolish" after all. They're as real as a heart attack (in every sense). In fact, maybe having anxiety, panic attacks, or stage fright makes more sense than *not* having them. Maybe it's the anxious ones, maybe even the panickers, who are the normal ones. Maybe my body—and maybe yours, too—has been doing exactly what it was designed to do all along.

These findings offered me massive relief. For years I believed I was the recipient of some cruel kink in the human genome—a mutation that I had no choice but to keep secret. What evolutionary biologists and psychologists helped show me was that anxiety—and, for me, occasions of panic—did not mean I was broken beyond repair. Yes, sometimes mental shit happened. But it wasn't the result of a system error built into the CPU in my skull. My body and brain were actually working as they were designed to.

This knowledge helped me stop hating my mind for its unpredictability and instead begin to marvel at the powers it can harness. I had brokered an uneasy truce with my brain. But understanding the principle of my mind's smoke detector didn't mean I couldn't also do my best to better calibrate it. It was time to start journeying toward the end of panic.

CHAPTER 5

Disclosure

Flying Southwest Airlines is like online dating. It offers self-seating only, which makes walking down the economy-only aisle something of a swipe-right-or-left experiment. Everyone ends up sizing up everybody else: *He's eating a tuna sub, pass. This one has sooo many bags on their lap, pass. This one looks desperate to talk someone's ear off, BIG pass.*

On a December evening in late 2020, I stalked one of those aisles, stinking of failure, sniffing for a place to lick my wounds.

As in life, you tend to get what you need on a Southwest flight, but not always what you think you want. I spotted an aisle seat next to a gentle-looking middle-aged woman knitting at the window, so I sat down, hoping her knitting would yield some scalp-tingling ASMR and a bit of comfort.[*]

---

[*] ASMR stands for "autonomous sensory meridian response." It's a tingly feeling that experts say about 20 percent of people experience when hearing such sounds as whispering, the crinkling of gift wrap, or the swish of a paintbrush across a canvas (contributing to my childhood devotion to PBS landscape painter Bob Ross). There are massive subgenres of ASMR online, and professional performers who make boatloads of money for their whispering skills.

Problem was, before I could zone out to her handiwork, curiosity took over. She was working the yarn in a way I'd never seen, with unfamiliar-looking needles. So I asked her about it and conversation flowed—that natural exchange of information humans are so good at. She told me her name was Cat and that she used to be a nurse, now in medical compliance. This was during the peak of Covid—and we found there was much for us to talk about, not least that Cat had become a Covid "long-hauler." She was flying to LA from Georgia to visit her daughter and grandbaby for the holidays. When she politely asked what I'd been doing in Arizona, I unloaded the whole miserable story.

I had traveled to Phoenix to cover the first major practice run of Pfizer's Covid vaccine rollout, filing segments for *Good Morning America* and *World News Tonight*. The end of my suspension in late February 2020 had more or less coincided with the outbreak of Covid-19, and toward the end of 2020 I'd reported almost exclusively on the subject for nearly eight months. Like so many reporters, I had become something of a lay expert on the matter.

Earlier that same day I'd spoken to a lawyer friend, describing to him my life with panic and telling him that I was thinking about sharing my struggles with others. I fretted about notifying ABC. I'll never forget his soaring, lawyerly retort: "My friend, ever heard of the Americans with Disabilities Act? They cannot fire you over that."

After the flash of relief—*"they cannot fire you"*—I was seized by a new thought. *Wait, do I have a disability?*

Hours later that question was still bouncing around in my brain as I loitered near my rental car while the crew was setting up our live shot. I figured I'd smoke a cigarette in the parking lot, like a high school kid hiding behind the gym. For some reason this Covid story felt like a good time to fall off the wagon; I'd already closet-smoked several cigarettes that day, hating myself with each inhale.

I walked back to where my producer and crew had set up our shot. Though I had spent months covering Covid and most of the previous twenty-four hours soaking up information from the hospital staff, though I knew the topic cold, and though I had been focused for months now on preventing panic, I felt failure brewing. I walked to the shot with the footsteps of the condemned, sensing a panic the way a parent uncannily predicts their kids' roughhousing will end in tears in precisely twenty-seven seconds.

Desperate to stave it off, I drew from my well-worn panic playbook. Now standing in front of the camera, I folded forward for toe touches and did some torso twists, the kind of light stretching said to help relieve tension in the back and also in the brain. Then I started chatting with the crew about something mundane. It was in the mid-60s and dry—snowbird dream weather—yet the familiar trickle of sweat dribbled down my spine. I thought for a moment about whether I had put on a lucky pair of underwear that morning. As the drumbeat of my pulse went from Muzak to death metal, I inventoried the amount of coffee I'd had that day. Couldn't remember, probably too much.

World News started. I listened to David Muir introduce my piece, with periodic countdowns from the director ahead of my live portion. At "forty-five seconds to the jump," I felt the elephant take her seat on my chest. I tried sucking in a few big gulps of air to avoid going hypoxic on camera. "Fifteen seconds to the jump," called the director. More air, then a quick smoothing of the typically unruly eyebrows. All of a sudden, I realized I'd forgotten how to swallow.

I can't swallow! How do I swallow?

"Five seconds . . ."

Thumpthumpthumpthump.

When Muir asked me our prearranged question about the vaccine's shelf life, I opened my mouth to speak. The words I'd painstakingly gathered into a couplet an hour earlier had scattered, as if blasted by a leaf blower. What came out was the sound I imagine a hen makes laying an egg: *Ehhhk.*

No! It's happening again!

In an eternity measured in milliseconds, my frontal lobe regained control and began frantically grabbing at random words blown about the landscape of my mind. Having not yet taken a breath, my vocal cords lumped syllables together, accruing into sentences. Their meaning was mostly the same as I had intended, but the polish and the confidence were gone.

As soon as it was over, I fled to the airport, lugging my carry-on and my shame hangover, determined to make the one flight that might get me home before the kids went to sleep. This panic had been especially dispiriting because, in the months since my suspension, I had been working—really working, for the first time—to put panic in the rearview mirror. I had nearly fooled myself into believing I had succeeded.

I was still playing a loop of the panic in slow-motion instant replay as I slid into seat 13C.

Maybe it was the mane of gray hair. Maybe it was the knitting. Maybe I had reached the breaking point. For whatever reason, I shed the mask of on-air perfection, giving Cat the unvarnished truth, laying out my panic the way I had never really done before, and certainly not with a stranger.

In return, Cat confided in me not just about her own trauma and troubles, but those of her daughter, whose emetophobia—the fear of choking or vomiting—was so severe that just seeing someone else gag could trigger panic attacks in her. I felt sympathy for Cat and her daughter. The two of us bonded over the way panic and anxiety had invaded our lives.

As we made our mutual disclosures, I could feel the weight of that latest panic lift ever so slightly off my shoulders. This kind of talking, I realized, was good medicine. Sitting next to Cat, I wondered: What are the odds that the first random person I fully opened up to about panic has also been so profoundly impacted by it?

In the coming months I would learn: the odds were good. It wasn't fate or a fluke that we connected over our shared experience surrounding panic. Nearly all of us have endured a once-in-a-lifetime attack, have panic disorder, or know someone else who does. Pretty soon people like this would become much more to me than the faceless statistics inhabiting the studies I'd been reading. These were real humans—some of whom, it turned out, I already knew.

SAFETY IN NUMBERS

I began testing the water with colleagues. During that first year of Covid, to avoid crowded airports and planes, our producer-reporter teams often elected to drive rather than fly. So we found ourselves with lots of time to talk. Passing through the badlands of northern Arizona on one of those drives, I confessed my panic to a producer in her twenties, the talented Lissette Rodriguez. As she drove and I rode shotgun, I clumsily danced around the topic until I finally came out with it. *Drum roll, please . . . Ahem.*

"Lissette, I have panic attacks. On air. They're bad."

Lissette: *Meh.*

More precisely, she said, "Oh, my sister also has panic attacks." Turns out it was no big deal for her. She said it was partly a generational thing—people her age just talk more openly about anxiety and panic. There's a lot less stigma about mental health issues for millennials than for Gen Xers like myself.

I was relieved, if mildly disappointed that my punch line had landed so softly. Hoping to elicit a burst of sympathy— *Oh, I would never have known! How terrible! All these years?!*—I amped up my delivery.

"Like, Lissette, really, these are full-blown meltdowns."

Another *meh*. What Lissette offered wasn't indifference— more like shrugging acceptance. She described matter-of-factly her sister's panics and how she deals with them. The conversation then flowed onward without awkwardness, despite my initial fumbling.[*]

I started telling more people in my professional orbit. Many did express surprise, including then ABC News' senior vice president of news gathering, Wendy Fisher, my longtime boss and friend. But her reaction was followed only by sympathy and acceptance, before the conversation with her, too, naturally meandered away toward a different topic.

All my hand-wringing seemed to be for naught. The firing squad I'd envisioned remained solely where it had been assembled: in my imagination. I started telling friends, and pretty much anyone with whom I'd engage in deep conversation—something I was starting to do much more often. It was shocking how many of them—millionaire businessmen, teachers, travel agents, and lawyers—told me they, too, had panic attacks.

Disclosure is, of course, one of the oldest and most primal forms of psychological relief. There is a reason my Roman

---

[*] Even when I called her a year later to ask if I might share this vignette, she remained blasé: "Oh, yeah. So many people in my family suffer from that. They often just say it's low blood sugar or something."

Catholic buddies growing up in New Jersey ducked into the confession booth weekly. It wasn't that their sins were so immense or novel; it was that unburdening provided them with psychological absolution. That's likely the reason why communal sharing—often in the form of group therapy, among people suffering the same or similar maladies—is so common and so successful.

If sharing with Cat, Lissette, and Wendy offered the beginnings of relief, could group therapy take me even further?

In the weeks after that flight with Cat, I hunted online for panic attack support groups. I found a blog titled exactly what I hoped to achieve: *Peace from Panic*. As I read the blog posts, I began to fully realize how many people's lives have been damaged by panic attacks, and how deeply—in ways often far more life-changing than mine. I decided to reach out to the site's author in hopes of learning more.

Like me, Jeni Driscoll had been battling panic for twenty years. She offered me some best practices for managing life with panic, as she'd collected them. As is so often the case, these strategies focused on the combination of therapies and pharmaceuticals that worked for her. She explained that, when she was in her twenties, her panics intensified and also came to include depersonalization and derealization (or DPDR). Supermarkets were her bête noire (this is much more common than you'd think). She told me she had studied broadcast journalism herself and had been inches away from hopping on a plane for her dream job at a Montana TV station. But partly because of her panic, she decided to stay in Southern California, where she married her sweetheart and eventually became a stay-at-home mom—not exactly the life she'd planned for, but a choice she says she doesn't regret.

In the months after our initial conversation, we checked in with each other. I'd always wondered about her decision not to get on that plane, so I finally asked her about it. Eventually, she told me, "I was thankful I didn't take that job in Montana and didn't pursue a career in journalism, because I wondered how I would ever have done that, especially being live on camera, when I felt panicky. As much as I missed the news business, I felt maybe it was for the best. Later, I did some work as a private investigator, which I loved because I could use my interviewing/writing/reporting skills I learned for a career in journalism. Yet I didn't have to worry about being on camera and having a panic attack." Her comments resonated with me for all the obvious reasons.

The tagline of the blog she would go on to create reads: "Embracing, advocating and discovering happiness in mental health." She had put her emotions out there in a courageous way. Yet in the early years of her blog, this champion of panickers and the agoraphobic withheld something elemental: her name. She published anonymously, even after winning acclaim for her writing. It wasn't until late 2020, just weeks before we first spoke, that Jeni Driscoll had attached her real name to the site for the first time. It was liberating, she said: a public confession of the secret she'd long been hiding.

After speaking with Jeni, I was even more determined to find a therapy group close to my home. Real people I could connect with. So I waded into the thickets of the internet. To my surprise, I found no active panic attack support groups in Los Angeles, either virtual or in person. That seemed strange. Obviously, lots of people were affected by panic. I wondered why others weren't clamoring to found such groups—especially during the depths of the pandemic.

I widened my search, finding some promising leads on Facebook. I joined a couple of the site's groups devoted to panic and anxiety. They were hardly calming, though. Most had members posting desperate SOSs in the midst of their crises, or else paeans to the latest drug. There were lots of questions about SSRIs and benzos, and the side effects people felt from those drugs, as well as anger at doctors who either refused to prescribe such medications or ignored their nasty side effects. There were textbooks worth of self-diagnoses, or requests for a crowdsourced diagnosis—even some pleas for money to help agoraphobic people make it through the week or month. What I found, in short, was a catalog of human suffering that ran to thousands of pages.

Since this was the internet, everything posted on those pages lives on in perpetuity. In most cases, cries for help just dangled there for a while, with a gentle or informative comment or two coming only much later. The woman who wrote, "I hate my life," and whose panic attacks had caused her to "have the shakes inside my head and it burns up my face," had to wait a couple of days before another human responded: "trust me you're not alone i suffer every single day."

Another person posted: "I'm having a panic attack and I'm 13 weeks pregnant. I haven't had a panic attack in 8–9 months. I've been fine. I'm freaking out. It feels like a heart attack. idk ☺ I'm just scared." Three days later someone wrote back: "how are you now, prayers."

These support groups seemed less a place of comfort and more a dungeon of distress. They started to freak me out. They offered the gift of confession, of unburdening, but not the cushion of real human support on the other side. I posted a message to the board asking moderators if there were virtual rooms where actual humans could talk to one another. The moderator responded that, with permission, one is allowed to message a specific person, but never the group at large, adding, "We don't do personal."

Another visitor chimed in asking about Zoom meetings. The moderator's response was that of a harried parent being pestered by a child: "We do not allow Zoom meetings." A few of the group members jumped in asking why. The moderator replied, "We tried to, but a specific person unfortunately ruined that for everyone. So that will not be allowed here either. —Admin."

Duly chastened, my fellow group members and I retreated back to our keyboards. I tried the other panic groups I had joined. All to no avail. "So what do people do, where do they go if they want to find a support group, where they can talk to people when they are not in crisis?" I ventured in one instance. No reply from the administrator, but a fellow poster commented, "If you find this out, please let me know, too. I reached out to groups exactly for this reason. Thank you."

The internet wasn't giving me the easy answer I sought. But now I had a mission, and a constituency of more than one in need of help.

I turned to the good folks at the National Alliance on Mental Illness. Over a period of several months of queries, I came away empty-handed. So I tried the Anxiety and Depression Association of America, and they eventually sent me a list with dozens of entries for support groups dealing with various issues. But only *five* groups nationwide listed panic as one of their topics. Two of those were operated by laypeople who had formed a support network of their own, and both of those groups became pandemic casualties. One met for the last time on March 11, 2020, just as Covid-19 began its dominance over our lives. Minutes posted online from that meeting show a single attendee. The second, run by a Boston-based life coach named Doreen Menelly, met for fifteen years until Covid came. Over the years, Menelly told me, the costs of renting a room had been significant but surmountable. What couldn't be overcome was going virtual. When they started Zoom or FaceTime meetings, attendees started dropping out. Menelly says attendees became self-conscious; they could see themselves on-screen, which exacerbated their anxiety. Members of the defunct group communicate only sporadically now, by email alone.

All this was perplexing to me. One would think there would be a massive constituency for these types of groups. Even if you count only the narrowest category—Americans suffering from full-fledged panic disorder this calendar year— that's still more than ten million people. About as many as the population of Sweden. So where were they finding relief?

BLAME FREUD

Undeterred, I pestered the American Psychological Association next. They quickly and wisely offloaded me on their chief science officer, the aforementioned psychology professor, author, and all-around mensch Mitch Prinstein. When I mentioned how few panic support groups seemed to be out there, Prinstein told me he thought he could find something for me. A couple of months later, after his own queries, he confirmed what I had by then suspected: "I still haven't heard of one. You are exactly right."

I don't get it, I told Prinstein. For support with alcoholism, there are over 123,000 AA groups worldwide, there are over 14,000 Al-Anon groups in the United States and Canada, but only a handful of panic groups operate in the US?

It's an endemic problem, he suggested. "You can't see depression, you can't see a panic attack," he said. And in the United States, at least, you can't fix what you can't see. That's because, he explained, "Medicare, health care, health care professionals, health care insurance companies, they don't reimburse as much for [support] groups because it's not deemed to be as efficacious."

It would be easy to blame the big insurance companies. But they didn't start this, Prinstein suggests. Freud did. Well, sort of.

"Unfortunately, the way that psychology and psychiatry got started, through Freud, attached a lot of personal blame or early trauma to things," Prinstein said. "We don't believe in any of that now. But the field started with people embarrassed to talk about what symptoms they were experiencing, because it was thought that somehow [it implied] unconscious desires." Think the ick factor of the Oedipus complex.

In other words, psychology had the double helix of shame and secrecy embedded in its very DNA. Early treatment centers for mental illness became "really secretive and in some ways really inhumane," Prinstein said. It was as if mere mention of the malady would conjure up its evil spirit.

By the 1990s and 2000s, in the epoch of Oprah, discussing anxiety and mental illness had become far more acceptable. Yet panic remained obscure. That's partly because, as we've seen, panic attacks and panic disorder are so underdiagnosed. It also has to do with the nature of panic attacks themselves: assuming that someone can even name their affliction as "panic," often the last thing they'll want to do is speak about it publicly.

The stigma is hard to shake. Social perceptions are sticky things, passed down the generations like cleft chins or freckles. Just after graduate school, Prinstein did clinical rotations on panic disorder. He said that often he and other clinicians had to reframe the way patients thought about their mental health, trying to convince them to view panic "almost like [they] would see diabetes," he said.

Prinstein lamented the enormous gap between government spending on physiological medicine vs. psychological medicine. Most Americans, he says, will remember the fifteen-minute dental hygiene intervention they got in kindergarten, which has helped prevent tooth decay and cavities in generations of children. "Where is the fifteen-minute intervention to stop emotional dysregulation, depression, suicidality, anxiety, substance use?" he asked. "We don't build in mental health prevention into the school curriculum at all."

This helps explain why, even though we might cognitively grasp, when told by an ER physician, that we've suffered a *panic* attack, not a *heart* attack, we still struggle to override the subconscious scream telling us we're not just panicking, we're dying.

TUESDAYS WITH WORRY

At last, after months of searching, I found a therapy group—2,500 miles from home. Headed by a psychologist who specializes in panic, the group used to meet in person, in Brooklyn, but Covid forced them to convert to virtual. So they opened their Zoom windows to people like me and other fellow travelers living across the continent hungry for community. It included panic sufferers from California, Washington, Chicago, Michigan, Boston, and Rhode Island. There were so many people in the first session I attended that it took over forty minutes just to get through the session's introductions.

Knowing that my turn to speak was coming up, I began to feel the familiar pangs of anxiety. This was the first time I'd joined a support group of any kind, and I was trying to formulate a couple of sentences that would not sound overwrought. Not only was I nervous, I was embarrassed for feeling nervous. Here, of all places, I should feel comfortable revealing myself.

At last, with a touch of a tremble in my voice, I did a version of the spiel I'd watched people do countless times on film or TV.

"Hi, my name is Matt, I live in Los Angeles, and I am a TV news correspondent who gets panic attacks on TV."

Secrets make loners. With this group, at least, I no longer had a secret. In one specific way, I belonged among the assembly of small, pixelated squares populating my iPad. Some people came on as amorphous voices, named tiles reluctant to show their faces. Others opted for those machine-generated Zoom backgrounds. But they were all people to some degree like me. It was a relief to be in their company.

For all the comfort it offered, though, I have to admit it also shook me. It was the first time, in the twenty-plus years since my first nut-kick of panic, that I was able to hear others with panic disorder tell their own stories en masse. Some experienced similar symptoms of the "courageous coward." One was a college student, a stage actor who never experienced a shred of fear while performing before hundreds of audience members but who wilted in common social situations or, like so many others, at the supermarket.

To some, the fear of a panic attack was so paralyzing that it overwhelmed their ability to perform almost any "normal" activity. Many were locked in a hopeless loop of agoraphobia. In order to drive a car, those with driving phobias described having actual safety blankets and ice packs (to cool their panicked sweating) riding shotgun with them. Sometimes, in conquering one fear, members gained a new one. A brave soul living in Staten Island managed to conquer his fear of driving over bridges—something that's hard to avoid when you live in an island borough in New York City. But on an extended drive around the five boroughs, he encountered the city's major tunnels, which triggered panic and a new phobia.

I quickly realized how little my episodes of panic had inhibited my life, at least when compared to my fellow attendees. I had a family and a steady job, a house, kids, two dogs, and a cat. Some of the people in those Zooms were alone in the world—fear of panic had made them so reclusive they couldn't see friends. Think about what it must be like to have your daily decisions weighed down with a thousand pounds of fear, knowing that talking to a stranger, checking out at the supermarket, driving to work, eating at a restaurant—any of it could trigger panic.

I had spent months learning about the way my social-rejection-induced panic made sense when viewed through an evolutionary lens. No, I was not likely to die from expulsion like our tribal ancestors might have, but I could easily lose my job, be cast out into the wilderness of the unemployed, weakening my family's financial security. The panic-inducing scenarios that set most of my fellow group members trembling, however, weren't nearly as abstract as mine.

Take several of the group members' fear of driving. Who doesn't know someone killed in a car crash? When I was a child, my parents had to take me to a psychologist to work through my recurring nightmare that they would die in a fiery wreck one night on a road we frequently traveled about a mile from our home. Indeed, motor vehicle crashes are the leading cause of death for Americans from ages one to fifty-four, making us the most murderous drivers in the developed world. If we drove as well as (or less badly than) drivers in other developed countries, 18,000 American lives would be saved every year. So maybe it makes sense that some folks' brains register driving as a mortal threat, one that could provoke a panic attack.

Something similar could be said for fear of flying, another

common phobia. Yes, the statistics indicate driving is far deadlier, but think about it: hurtling at 500 miles per hour in an aluminum tube seven miles in the air, packed with other germ-spewing humans, seems positively bonkers. Even agoraphobia makes a kind of sense: your home is a place of safety, the domain of near-absolute control; everything outside is the realm of chaos, danger, and disease (not to mention traffic accidents).

In our group, sealed off from the judgment of society, my fellow panickers could talk openly about what they called their "craziness." The depth of their pain was a revelation, but so was the height of their courage in talking about it.

In the months that followed, the group spawned a subgroup that met on the weeks the main Brooklyn-based psychologist took off. Eventually a couple of us created a WhatsApp group, offering an additional haven to chat, encourage, and vent in real time. It was a place where real people could tap out a text, but also call anyone at any time, where they shared pictures of their successes (often involving travel) and sources of joy (so often kids and pets).

Among the core WhatsApp group's founders was a man I'll call Mark, who also lived in California. Mark is handsome, with sleeve tattoos and the impossibly dense beard of a movie villain. When he wasn't flying planes for fun—with his adorable family inside—his job as an airport operations manager was to ensure that planes didn't crash into each other and to prevent unwelcome guests (or lunatics) from storming the airfield.

Mark shared with me his own panic origin story. He'd experienced a freakish streak of death when he was younger— a family member hit by a truck, a friend killed by a stray bullet, another friend who died by suicide. It messed with his internal gyroscope. His first panic attack happened right on cue, when he was eighteen or nineteen. He'd been having headaches, so he went to a doctor to have his brain scanned. When he called for the results, it seemed the receptionist was upset and hung up on him brusquely. That short exchange sent him into a panic spiral: *The receptionist must know I have a fatal brain tumor.* Panic symptoms washed over him. Finally, bathed in doom and sweat, he willed his trembling fingers to dial the doctor's office again, pumping the receptionist for the painful truth.

"It's a tumor, right? I'm dying?"

"What? No!" She explained that the doctor would have to call him, but no, he was totally fine. She'd just been in a rush. Nothing to worry about.

He may have been cancer-free, but his panic was there to stay. Over the years it would kick up around major milestones and decisions. He was so fearful of panicking in public, his biggest secret spilling out for the world to see, that for a time he became borderline agoraphobic. He could tolerate the shopping aisles of the supermarket, but not the checkout line, because the cashier might notice the twitching in his face—see what he called the "scared kitten in the grown man"—and that split second of perceived judgment could set him off. He told me there were times he couldn't even climb the stairs at home "without my heart freaking out."

It was just before the birth of his first child that Mark decided, after years of attempting to manage anxiety and panic through meditation and therapy, to try medication. He has been on Lexapro, a drug indicated for depression and anxiety, for over four years, and he swears they've been the most stable years of his life. (Some antidepressants have been found to provide the off-label bonus of reducing the incidence of panic, though no one's sure how, or why they work for some, like Mark, and not others, like me.)* He told me he hasn't suffered from panic since. The resulting stability enabled his marriage and career to flourish.

Mark told me he found our panic support group as eye-opening as I did—especially the duration of some of the members' panic-induced agoraphobia. During one of our talks he reminded me of the time a homebound member of our Whats-App group reported that she'd gone to the supermarket. It was apparently one of the few times she'd left the house since Covid-19 emerged. That step—an insignificant chore for many of us, a milestone for her—was met with a barrage of hearts and cheers. It was exactly the kind of social support that many of us had been missing for years.

FULL CIRCLE

I knocked on the door of a bungalow-style home in Ventura County, California. Through the window, I saw a woman in the kitchen with her back to me. All I could make out was her thick gray hair. She disappeared for a second, then opened the door, and we fell into an embrace as natural as our first conversation. And she held me for a long time. As we stepped back from the embrace I realized it was the first time I had seen Cat's entire face. It had been a little over a year since our intimate conversation on the Southwest plane from Phoenix to Los Angeles. We had exchanged emails and texts since, but we had been masked on that flight. We'd only seen each other's eyes.

Now at the home of her daughter Ayla and son-in-law Andrew, Cat proudly ushered me to the living room, where

---

* And yes, I've also tried Lexapro, but it caused nasty side effects in me, so my doctor discontinued it.

Ayla was on the carpet bottle-feeding one of their two adopted children, just eight months old. Ayla had dangling curls and deep-set brown eyes. Her toddler was in a princess dress, spinning and hopping in imitation of the ballerinas skittering across the stage in the Bolshoi's thundering version of the *Nutcracker* playing on a big-screen TV.

Ayla and I had been in touch during the previous six months, too, talking about her panic and emetophobia. First we spoke on the phone; it was late at night and Ayla was exhausted from caring for her recently adopted toddler (the ballerina). A few days later she wrote me an email, taking another crack at explaining her emetophobia and the panic it produces.

"What happens when I suspect or see someone vomit: Time seems to slow down. I feel a sense of dread and horror. Thoughts are impossible; I am reduced to a flight instinct. My body shakes, my breathing is fast and shallow, my heart is pounding. Basic adrenaline response. Senses are heightened—that's why I close my eyes and ears, otherwise I am completely honed in on the ill person and every movement and sound they made is imprinted in my brain. I can vividly recall nearly every instance of someone vomiting in front of me, though what happened before or after, that I couldn't tell you."

Ayla could sense that this kind of reaction was unusual when she noticed others, like her husband, barely register when a diner at a nearby table had a coughing fit—the kind of thing that might cause her to have a panic and flee a restaurant. She told me she began to avoid "cruises, boat trips, car trips with anyone outside of my family whose motion sickness propensity I do not know, public bathrooms, playgrounds, amusement parks, restaurants (and specific foods—I do not eat much seafood and rarely eat salads because of the risk of food poisoning), flying, and traveling in general." This was the clearest description I'd seen of how phobias that trigger panic attacks can bloom into agoraphobia.

It required a great deal of accommodation and work, but in the early years of her marriage to Andrew she got her emetophobia more or less under control. But when Ayla wanted to have a baby, her life became like the trials of Job. She had multiple miscarriages and finally an ectopic pregnancy, which is when the egg is fertilized outside the uterus, a condition that can be deadly. One of the main symptoms of ectopic pregnancy happens to be her biggest fear: constant nausea. She began to question God. "I used to easily label myself a Christian, but I identify now as agnostic," she told me. "I don't know what sort of higher power would see fit to fuck me over with this phobia and anxiety and then let me experience multiple miscarriages and an ectopic pregnancy with paralyzing nausea."

She lost that baby and gave up on having a child of her own, but not on being a mother. She and her husband decided to adopt. And *of course* the baby they adopted, who became that twirling three-year-old in the princess dress, would be a puker. But they got through it and, mustering monumental courage, decided to adopt again.

Given Ayla's description of her chaotic life, I expected to see a frazzled family in an upturned house when I arrived that afternoon in Ventura. Instead, Ayla projected almost as much calm as her mother (and her house was immaculate).

We chatted, and she told me about her last major panic. It had happened about six months earlier, when Ayla had gotten a call from her daughter's school. "Your daughter threw up," she was told. "Could you come pick her up?" A routine-enough call for your typical preschool teacher, but a five-alarm fire for Ayla. Plus, this particular call came as she was in the midst of both finding a new home *and* fostering a third child.

"Okay, we'll come in just a minute," she told the teacher as casually as she could. But internally she was exploding. "I just fucking lost my mind. I was imagining all these kids I now had were going to get norovirus, and that we all were going to get norovirus.* I know it sounds ridiculous, but I just was imagining all three of these children that I already was over my head with—all just puking everywhere, and I was shaking. I could not stop shaking."

Ayla had been driving when she got the call, and she began obsessively running her hands through her hair, bouncing her legs, feeling waves of nausea come over her. The nausea only amplified her panic. Fortunately, Cat was with her and urged Ayla to pull over so that she could take the wheel. "She didn't even pull over in a safe place," Cat remembered. "She just stopped on the side of the road, like, 'Okay, this is gonna have to be good enough.'" When they got home with her daughter, Ayla retreated to her room and took a benzo to calm down.

Then she had a thought: Maybe her daughter *hadn't* contracted norovirus. Maybe they wouldn't all spend the week puking. Maybe it was a urinary tract infection or some other, more common, nonfatal bug that kids routinely get?

She roused herself and took her daughter to the emergency room, just to check. As a nurse conducted an exam, her daughter threw up again, the vomit splattering on Ayla's shoes. But it didn't trigger the panic she feared it might. She handled it.

From the vantage point of a few months, Ayla assessed the episode. She explained that reframing the incident in her head, coupled with a well-timed dose of antianxiety medi-

---

* A massively contagious virus that causes vomiting and diarrhea.

cine, had changed everything. As the *Nutcracker*'s Mouse King bounced on the big screen behind her, Ayla confided in me that the episode had prompted her to reconsider her choice to adopt the third child she had been fostering. It was a hard decision, forgoing the chance to love and protect another small child, but also, ultimately, a massive relief. She said she hadn't suffered a major panic since.

When it was time to leave, Cat, still in her socks, padded out into the street to walk me to my car. I told her that, just as Ayla had managed to change her outlook, Cat had helped me change mine. She helped destigmatize my panic. It was no longer the stain I had to rub out, no longer a source of shame. In that sense, I had come quite a long way.

There was still a long way to go. I thought about the moments immediately after a car crash. You sit there staring at your crumpled hood and the first thing your brain registers is its very consciousness: *Okay, I'm alive.* (Woo-hoo!) Next comes a mental pat-down: an assessment of possible limbs broken, joints tweaked, innards rejiggered.

That was where I stood. I knew that panic was natural, I knew my body was working as it should, I knew there was no reason for me to be ashamed. I now also knew panic could do a number on a person's health. I had no sense what kind of damage twenty years of near-daily hormonal car crashes might have caused my brain and body. It was time to look under the hood.

CHAPTER 6

When the Doctor Sees You

By now I had done enough late-night Google doom-searches, and backed them up with enough interviews with luminaries in the field, to be fully freaked out about the harm anxiety and panic inflict on the body. The National Institutes of Health's PubMed database lists nearly 300,000 studies on anxiety, many of which detail its negative impact on physiological health. Chronic anxiety can increase blood pressure and the concomitant risk of heart disease. It can trash your digestive system, cause diarrhea and constipation, and ruin your gut flora, and has been associated with irritable bowel syndrome.

It's not only the "basket cases" who are affected: "Even with low levels of psychological distress—certainly much lower levels than would attract a diagnosis of anxiety or depression—these people had an increased risk of mortality from all causes," reported one study. Social rejection—a form of which I felt after a panic—is apparently particularly poisonous. The APA's Mitch Prinstein elaborated: "It leads to depression and inflammatory disease. Social rejection increases the risk of premature death by 100 percent, which is slightly higher than the risk of premature death from twenty or more cigarettes a day. So our social rejection can hurt us more than being a chronic smoker." It ruins quality of sleep, which can further distort judgment and cause hormonal dysregulation. Studies testing the impulse control of socially rejected (mostly young) people indicate that they are more likely to do harmful things to others when feeling rejected or isolated. It's little wonder that a meta-survey found that the vast majority of school shooters felt socially rejected.

The more I learned about the physiological impact of my panic and anxiety, the more convinced I became that, across the decades, they had raised hell on my brain and organs. I felt a sudden urgency to make an appointment with my general practitioner, if just to assess the depth of the damage before I began focusing in earnest on remedies.

A few weeks later I sat in front of his broad oak desk. Dr. Kamran Rabbani wears a lab coat and actually takes time listening to his patients. When I explained why I was there and requested more or less every test he had, he looked up from his notepad. Perhaps because of the desperate way I described my panic, or the fact that I hadn't similarly imposed on him before, he took me seriously. He ordered up four kinds of blood tests, a urine analysis, and something called a "cerebrovascular profile carotid and vertebral duplex scan." I had no idea what that was, but I liked how serious it sounded.

When the tests were completed, Dr. Rabbani called me at 8:00 p.m. one evening, long after his office hours. He started by saying he didn't want to wait until morning to talk to me.

This was not an encouraging sign.

"Do you drink a lot of water?" he asked.

I swallowed hard. "Yes . . . ?" I braced myself.

"Okay, I want you to eat more pickles or salty foods. Your

sodium is low." He also wanted me to get more sun, because my vitamin D levels were a touch low. Save for those things, nearly every single test was normal.

"You're extremely healthy," he exclaimed.

"What about my cortisol?" I asked. Anxiety and panic are supposed to spike your cortisol, to damaging effect.

"Well," he said, "it's nothing to worry about. It was actually on the low side of normal."

My cortisol levels were *low*?

The news was comforting, though a little baffling—even disappointing. How could a person who had endured multiple panics a week for the better part of a decade, whose stress levels were through the roof, be so seemingly robust? It seemed to defy conventional wisdom, not to mention so much of what I had been reading. Could my pathetic meditation practice have been the key? Was it exercise? Diet?

It could be any one of those things, a combination, or none at all, according to Dr. Isaac Gardner. A psychoneuro-endocrinologist, he studies the connection between hormones and human behaviors. Gardner explains that, while counter-intuitive, low cortisol levels in people who should seemingly have high resting cortisol levels is normal. "It's probably protective," he says, "because the body adjusts to the stress." He suggests that, evolutionarily, early human hunter-gatherers were exposed to constant life-or-death stress and that perpetually high cortisol levels would probably have killed them. So they adapted. The successful ones—who would end up breeding more surviving babies—likely evolved, he said, "to downregulate that system, so that our cortisol would be lower even if we are responding to a lion attack all the time."

I also enjoy multiple antidotes to social rejection: a spouse, children, family and friends. Now, with access to a panic group, there were only more people who could offer me support. All of those factors significantly mitigate the possible physical harm of regular spikes of cortisol.

Also, Gardner put an end to another fear: that all those years of war zones, natural disasters, and panic attacks had depleted my natural store of adrenaline. That supposed depletion is popularly referred to as "adrenal fatigue." One of the most prolific lay diagnosticians I knew, my mother—for whom accuracy was secondary—had been convinced for a decade that I indeed suffered "adrenal fatigue."

At this point Gardner nearly yelled into the phone with frustration: "You do not run out of hormones because of chronic stimulation of them—that's nonsense. There are people who have adrenal insufficiency . . . that's an autoimmune disease, and you don't have that!"

In other words, when it came to accrued health effects of my panic, the experts were telling me to chill out.

TEMPLE

As I sought out further insight and guidance, my journey into managing panic approaching its next phase, I turned to luminaries beyond medicine. One of them was Dr. Temple Grandin, among the world's foremost experts on how animals experience the world. I had originally reached out to her to ask whether humans were unique in suffering panic attacks. The professor of animal behavior at Colorado State University and prolific author explained that certain animals experience tonic immobility, like chickens and fainting goats. Cattle suffer nearly the same spectrum of symptoms as panicking humans when they're separated from their herd (often preceding a one-way trip to the slaughterhouse).

The conversation flowed from the animal perspective on panic to the human perspective, something in which Grandin has intimate knowledge.

Grandin grew up not speaking much. Before autism became better understood, she was considered a developmentally "stunted" child. Some doctors thought she might have suffered brain damage. Much has changed in the decades since, both in our understanding of autism and for Grandin herself. Today, the renowned scientist and animal behaviorist is based in northern Colorado and favors western shirts buttoned to the top and cinched with a bolo tie. The same person who grew up barely talking as a child is now a feted public speaker with a voice as melodic as a country song.

Two minutes into our first conversation, she asked me if I'd tried antidepressants. I told her I had been taking Paxil for many years and that it had been useful in reducing my generalized anxiety, if not my panic. She told me that for years she, too, had had panic attacks, spent hours frozen in fear as if her "nervous system was hyped for living in a jungle with dangerous animals." This was in the early 1980s. And because she is who she is, she was determined to find a solution. She started living in the library, devouring clinical studies about antidepressants. She took her findings about these then-new drugs to her doctor and convinced him to prescribe them to her.

Antidepressants were key to Grandin's stability and ultimately, she told me, to her success in life. She's been on desipramine for forty years.

Grandin is friendly but direct as a mule kick. "If you have been on Paxil for more than fifteen years, I recommend *not* going off of it," she told me. "I repeat, *not* going off it, because I've seen a lot of people on [it], and I'd be willing to bet, especially if you've been on it for that long, that it's probably doing a lot more for you than you think it is."

"Well," I responded, "they say these antidepressants should not be 'forever drugs.'"

"Uh-uh," she answered skeptically. "I know a guy who went off Prozac, and let me tell ya, he's paying the price for it . . . It's very bad."

This went on for a bit. Grandin sang the praises of just the right dose of an antidepressant, noting that hers had cured her of physical ailments, panic, insomnia, and more. It saved her life. "It was ninety percent biochemistry. Better living with chemistry, for me," she said.

Grandin happened to have more appreciation for my experience doing TV news than I could have imagined. One of her friends, back in the 1980s, owned a six-foot satellite dish. At the time, it was capable of capturing the live satellite feeds that TV news teams beamed into control rooms in New York.* "We thought it was real good giggles to get the live news feeds before they officially went on air," she recounted in one of our conversations.

Many such giggles were generated by watching correspondents prep for their live reports. If you've ever watched Rafael Nadal prepare for a serve, you would understand: first the Spanish tennis great unlocks a wedgie in his butt, then loosens the sleeve of each arm, pulls his nose, tucks his hair back behind each ear, tugs on his nose again, leans forward, and bounces the ball ten to twelve times. Many reporters have their own versions of that.

---

* We no longer use satellite trucks beaming information to orbiting satellites. More commonly, TV news uses transmitters that aggregate signal from multiple cell phone SIM cards to send video.

"We would watch these news personalities do these weird things," she went on. "Oh, we would laugh at some of them."

So Grandin was one of the few people I'd met who wasn't in the news business but who had witnessed the whole "icing the kicker" phenomenon—correspondents prepping and practicing their lines during the interminable wait before they are called upon to perform. She said she could always see the little screwups they made when they actually went live.

Having seen my ilk in action, she assured me: "You. Can't. Be. Perfect."

HAPPY PILLS

In one of our conversations, I mentioned to Grandin that I had been reading about the promise of psychedelics. Researchers were putting out studies on neuroplasticity—in particular, the ability of certain hallucinogens, when coupled with "integration" (talk therapy), to change the way our brains are wired. Antidepressants seemed to numb painful symptoms; hallucinogens, it was increasingly said, seemed to offer a cure to mental health conditions.

But psychedelics and SSRIs do not play nicely together; antidepressants can interfere with the psychedelic experience. In some cases, they evidently trigger something called serotonin syndrome, which can be fatal.

At seventy-five, Grandin knows a thing or two. When she talks, you listen. She has persevered through tremendous challenges, and she's no stranger to mental illness. Each time we spoke, she urged me to be careful in my pursuit of an answer to panic attacks and, above all, to stay on my antidepressant. (My notes about our conversations are topped with a single question: "How many times did Temple tell me NOT to go off SSRIs?") She observed that my loved ones could probably evaluate an SSRI's impact on me better than I could. It's true: my wife always has this uncanny ability to intuit when I've forgotten to bring my meds with me on a longer trip. I arrive home feeling fluey and edgy, invariably prompting the question, "Did you forget your happy pills again?"

Over the years I had become convinced that "happy pills" were the chemical lifesaver keeping my sanity afloat. But in the aftermath of my suspension and the crisis of confidence it inspired, they didn't seem like enough anymore, especially because the meds failed to treat what seemed my mind's most urgent need: to kill the panic.

I knew enough already to be skeptical about SSRIs. No one was sure how or why they worked, how effective they were, or why they worked for some people and not for others. It wasn't until July 2022, over a year after those conversations with Grandin, that a groundbreaking study appeared confirming how wrong we might all have been about these serotonin boosters. Like, *really* wrong: "Our comprehensive review of the major strands of research on serotonin shows there is no convincing evidence that depression is associated with, or caused by, lower serotonin concentrations or activity."

The article, published in *Molecular Psychiatry,* went on to detonate the long-peddled notion that "chemical imbalances" cause depression and certain mood disorders. Medical professionals, operating in good faith on the science they had access to, had advanced a chemical imbalance theory—suggesting that our mood disorders were the consequence of a disturbance in our natural brain chemicals. The public duly absorbed this notion, "leading to a pessimistic outlook on the outcome of depression and negative expectancies about the possibility of self-regulation of mood." What's worse, the chemical imbalance theory of depression "may discourage people from discontinuing treatment, potentially leading to lifelong dependence on these drugs."

That's not all. The article also asserted that SSRIs were potentially dangerous to patients. They can be much more addictive than patients have been told, and withdrawal symptoms from the medications can be significant.

Psychiatrist Ellen Vora, author of *The Anatomy of Anxiety,* has for many years collected anecdotal evidence that mirrors the results of the *Molecular Psychiatry* study. She calls patients' dependence on antidepressants, from SSRIs to benzos, "the silent epidemic." A big part of her personal practice in recent years, she told me, involves working with patients addicted to their happy pills.

Her patients often come to her with a near-identical story: They were going through a stressful time, so their doctor prescribed an antidepressant and their life stabilized. But "when they decided to get off of Lexapro, all hell broke loose. They're irritable, they can't sleep . . . some of them even become suicidal. And they don't know to attribute that to withdrawal. They just think, 'Wow, I really was depressed. I really needed Lexapro. It really was helping.' So then they go back on Lexapro, they feel instantly better, and they think to themselves, and I quote, because it's always the same story: 'Lexapro saved my life.' And what actually happened there is that nothing feels as good as scratching the itch of withdrawal with the withdrawn substance itself."

It's more than just dependence. Antidepressants come with gastrointestinal and sexual side effects, all of which, she says, should be part of a doctor's informed consent when prescribing these meds. When prescribed SSRIs, most of us are warned of sexual side effects and also weight gain. But addiction and withdrawal symptoms? Nope. In my sessions, it has never come up.

There's still more, and it's bad. Vora says it is possible that antidepressants may actually help *trigger* panic attacks in people like me. An antidepressant is most potent, she says, shortly after you swallow the pill. But the more time passes, the more your body metabolizes the drug—meaning your body is coming down from it and craving more. That period just before you take your regular dose again is when you might suffer "interdose withdrawal"—when your body craves its next hit. And that, explains Vora, "is a really ripe time to feel panicky. So depending on when people take their pill, they wake up [in the morning] in a panic or wake up in the middle of the night and panic."

For many psychiatrists Paxil is particularly unpredictable. ASU's Randy Nesse told me he used to prescribe Paxil more often but found it "had more side effects and was harder to get off than other agents." As for me, I took my Paxil in the evenings—in the hours after *World News Tonight* aired and my live shots for a given day were over. Could I have been suffering the kind of interdose withdrawal Vora described just as I went on air, exacerbating my tendency toward panic?

All this would come to light many months after my conversation with Temple Grandin. All I could say for certain in the moment was that conventional meds were not solving my most pressing mental health concern. No matter how fiercely Temple insisted I stick with my pills, I had to believe there was something more out there for me.

SLEDGEHAMMERS AND SAFETY BEHAVIORS

Of course, medication isn't the only remedy for panic. Nearly every one of the anxiety specialists I interviewed suggested cognitive behavioral therapy. CBT is widely considered the gold standard for treating panic. It was for this reason that in the spring of 2021 I made a pilgrimage to Austin to meet Dr. Michael Telch at the University of Texas's Laboratory for the Study of Anxiety Disorders. Telch is one of the world's preeminent specialists in CBT.

Sitting on the balcony of his townhouse overlooking Lake Austin, he referred to CBT as a "sledgehammer" treatment against panic. It has two main features. The first is psychoeducational: training a sufferer to recognize that panic is in their mind—purely a "mental distortion" (planes don't just fall out of the sky, supermarket cashiers are too busy to care about your twitchiness). Telch teaches panic patients that our triggers—vomit, a highway, the ding of armed doors on a plane—are actually harmless, and even the physical manifestations of a panic are not as catastrophic or debilitating as we believe.

The second element is exposure: gradually subjecting patients to the very thing they fear, whether it's driving, flying, going to the supermarket, or public speaking. Patient and practitioner work together to defang the phobia. It isn't Freud—there's no dwelling on one's past, no psychoanalyst's couch. CBT is super-practical and goal oriented. Telch told me he's cured patients in as few as two or three sessions.

When I described my pre–live shot rituals, hoping they might help me get through a panic, Telch gently explained that the calisthenics, smoking, air gulping, and magic underwear were classic "safety behaviors" and decidedly not constructive. In practice, he said, they only increased the chances of a panic. My "special preparations" were priming my mind to anticipate an encounter with a colossal threat, which only raised my anxiety levels. It was no surprise, he suggested, that panic often followed closely behind.

This made a lot of sense. I resolved to dial down my pregame rituals. (Note: this definitely helped.) The problem was, even after Telch's careful explanation, the basic tentpoles of CBT simply did not fully hold up in my case. If my on-air panic attack in January 2020 had taught me anything, it was that panic attacks *could* have real-world consequences. And, occasionally, planes do fall out of the sky (not a phobia I've ever had, but still). Such examples are a major reason why some psychologists criticize CBT for invalidating patients' phobias.

The second pillar was even trickier. I wondered what kind of exposures CBT experts might come up with that could replicate the real effect of a live shot. A few practitioners I spoke to tried their mightiest. "Well, I'd have you run up and down the stairs to raise your respiratory rate, and spin you in a desk chair to make you dizzy," said one, "and then have you present a live shot to me" (in his office). Others suggested they could tackle my social anxiety, and specifically fear of running afoul of my group, by forcing me to go to convenience stores and speak to store clerks or act silly in a restaurant.

I tried in vain to explain that I speak to strangers for a living, and that conditions for me to have a panic are nearly impossible to reproduce, short of ginning up a new TV news outlet with millions of loyal viewers and powerful execs watching from the control room. The doctors I spoke to generally insisted I was still thinking about the situation wrong, and that panic really was a trick of the mind that could be beat with a little of their trusty CBT.

Maybe I was being stubborn. Maybe I had gone through enough talk therapy and swallowed enough pills to be suspicious of what CBT or any conventional treatment could reasonably offer me. Maybe I wasn't feeling sufficiently heard by these doctors. Maybe I feared what it meant for my future if the "sledgehammer treatment" couldn't put a dent in my panic.

For whatever reason, I resisted going down the road of CBT. Presented with their offers, I kindly declined (for the time being). I had also begun to suspect, on a still-subterranean level, that my panic might be a presenting symptom of a larger malady, one that I hadn't yet unearthed and was harder to pinpoint.

It was around this time that, at my wife's behest, I started listening to podcasts focused on wellness. They tended to feature conventional-adjacent psychologists and experts like the holistic psychiatrist Ellen Vora. In hearing them speak, it became clear to me that, though it felt like I'd tried every tool in the toolbox, there were still a lot out there that I hadn't gotten even close to. Maybe I was too focused on topical solutions that couldn't penetrate the surface of my psyche—like slathering yourself in Neosporin to treat cancer.

I felt, in that moment, that I needed an altogether new approach, something that could treat "the whole human"—a salve that could seep into my core and heal me from within.

CHAPTER 7

Lobster Claws and Mushrooms

This may sound like the start of a Bruce Springsteen ballad. It's not quite. Back at my New Jersey high school, there was a football player named Lane Jaffe. Two grades above me, he was captain of both the football and lacrosse teams. An annoyingly effortless athlete, he won a scholarship to play lacrosse at Rutgers and starred all four years. In high school, Lane was one of the first to have facial hair, girlfriends, sex—things we underclassmen all desperately wanted. And in the days when hazing high school freshmen and sophomores was still tolerated, he had the distinction of being a nicer big man on campus than most.

Lane and I lost contact over the two decades since high school, but in the months before the pandemic began, he reached out, out of the blue. Turned out he was also living in LA. He was a yoga teacher now, with a devoted following, and he had started a promising breathwork practice. He'd battled what he called "depressive feelings" for years. Breathwork, peppered with psychedelics, had helped him find balance and wean off Wellbutrin. These days, even just a few years later, his pursuits are nearly ubiquitous in the wellness world, but when we started talking again in late 2019, he offered a message that felt both novel and persuasive.

As we eased back into friendship in the months that followed, Lane urged me to try breathwork. He'd spent about a year taking courses in LA and going on retreats in Costa Rica and Bali. He described the changes breathwork had had on his mind and even his physique. As a father with two kids whose incessant travel made him a homebody, I was initially reluctant. Plus, breathwork sounded too woo-woo for me, its promise of healing too far-fetched. So I put him off.

Suspension from your job does free up your schedule, though. So in early February 2020, I pulled up outside the Sanctum studio in Venice, California. From the outside, it looked like a hippie-chic junkyard (was that Ken Kesey and the Merry Pranksters' bus parked in the lot?). One Yelp reviewer described the place as "a vortex of love and beauty." Lane came out to greet me—bald head, light beard, intense dark eyes. He welcomed me with a bear hug and the familiar smell of home. He guided me into his studio, where ten or so people milled about waiting for class to begin. The room had vaguely arabesque decor and a large circular window, through which the January sun moseyed in. Lane handed me a yoga mat to lie on and a blanket to ward off the chill, adding that one can often feel cold during breathwork.

The technique he described seemed simple enough: two big breaths in through the mouth and one breath out of the mouth. Lane explained to the class that to achieve the most benefit, we had to breathe rapidly, like a piston: *two-in-one-out, two-in-one-out, two-in-one-out.*

He turned up the jungle beats on the speaker system and we started chugging air. Like a coxswain, Lane called out the cadence, pushing us to embrace the discomfort. I dove in, anticipating my reward would be something like the oozing goodness you feel after a yoga session or a massage. But all that mouth breathing led primarily to a deserty dryness in my mouth, as if every molecule of moisture had been vacuumed out. *Is everyone feeling this uncomfortable?* I wondered.

Lane kept pushing us. He later told me he noticed me "charging right out of the gate, breathing without fear." After about five minutes, I forgot about my mouth because my body had begun to shake. My hands and feet tingled and then went numb. After about fifteen minutes, he says, he noticed a smile on my face. I remember little of those early moments, aside from the strange feeling of my wrists curling inward, turning my hands into immobile lobster claws.

With my physical capacity gone, the emotion came. Quiet at first, it began to burble out. I was now sobbing, tears trickling into the little wells of my ears. It was rawer than sadness—this was pure, uncut pain. Lane came by, kneeling down and pressing his hands on my lower legs. He was letting me know that I was not alone. In the language of breathwork and psychedelics, he was "grounding" me, reconnecting me to the physical world.

He was not, however, trying to comfort me. As I would come to learn, pain is where the healing is. I let the emotion flow through me, unsure whether I actually wanted it to stop. Eventually Lane slowed the cadence for his breath-chugging crew and brought us into a relaxation meditation.

Intense breathwork like this is essentially deliberate hyperventilation. It's an extreme version of what happens to many people (unintentionally) during panic attacks, and it can amplify the symptoms of panic, including chest pain, lightheadedness, and anxiety. That's because by taking in *too much* air, you deprive your body of the carbon dioxide it needs to release oxygen into your system. That's the cruel irony of rapid breathing. Panickers will often overbreathe, thinking they need to in order to avoid hypoxia, but this only exacerbates the body's inability to uptake oxygen. The body reacts to oxygen deprivation by constricting blood vessels—thus the lobster claws. It's why breathing in a paper bag helps. By rebreathing your exhaled air, you're increasing the CO_2 in your lungs, and thus increasing your ability to intake oxygen. In the breathwork world, you *want* that shortage of CO_2. "Lobster claws" are a badge of honor, proof that you've "done the work."

Later Lane offered me a bit of further perspective. "It looked to me like a balloon that had filled up with so much air and the breathwork just allowed you to let out the pressure, to decompress. And you looked like you felt free from what you had been carrying around." It was a nice way to describe a grown man crying in a room full of strangers. Apparently this was normal in his classes. Lane says people have cried, laughed, even had orgasms during breathwork.

He was right. That relief stuck with me for weeks. I eagerly went back for a session a couple of weeks later, and again I geysered out sobs.

Then the pandemic hit, and the idea of joining a bunch of people clustered in a small room huffing their lungs out on one another seemed unwise. Sanctum would soon close its doors, and Lane, like the rest of the world, went virtual. I never joined any of those virtual classes. And truthfully, I probably wouldn't have ever become a regular attendee of "in real life" classes. The feeling of relief was profound, but so was the fear of getting caught in a gyre of grief and pain I could never escape.

Still, I recognized the truth of Lane's assessment: the deflating balloon that he saw in me was real. I could sense that it wasn't a little birthday balloon, either. This was a Hindenburg hovering within me, liable to burst into flames. It needed to be dealt with.

In our talks, I was attracted to what Lane told me about psychedelics, about the momentous change they had effected in him. I started doing some research of my own and found there was a growing body of evidence supporting their promise for people suffering from conditions like anxiety and depression. I was looking for a treatment that did more than alter the pace at which my brain's serotonin was emitted and absorbed, one pill at a time. Psychedelics seemed like they could hold the answer.

Ellen Vora, the psychiatrist who had introduced me to the concept of interdose withdrawal, told me that, by late 2020, psychiatric practitioners whose recommendations were confined to conventional meds, therapy, and CBT were "stuck five to ten years in the past." By now, Michael Pollan's book *How to Change Your Mind* had brought plant-based psychedelics into the public space. (It was part of the "cleanup work from the moral panic of the '60s and '70s," as Vora put it, referring to the stigma associated with such drugs in the aftermath of the federal government's clampdown on psychedelics.) She pointed to psilocybin, the chemical that makes the "magic" in certain species of mushroom and which she said was far less dangerous than alcohol and arguably less dangerous than many antidepressants.

As we approach the mid-2020s, said Vora, with characteristic pith, "I think that psychedelics are on the menu at this point. It's not such a wild ask of the waiter."

WHERE TO PLACE YOUR ORDER

As it turned out, I happened to share a bed with a patron who was placing just such an order. In the months after those breathwork sessions with Lane, my wife, Daphna, scheduled her own "guided mushroom journey." You have likely heard of microdosing. Maybe you've seen Hulu's *Nine Perfect Strangers*, in which Nicole Kidman's character runs a resort called Tranquillum House, where she slips her unwitting guests small (and eventually larger) doses of psilocybin. Microdoses—generally considered a tenth or less of a true "psychedelic" dose, which is 3.5 to 5.5 grams of psilocybin—are now so common in LA that folks will nibble a mushroom cap before yoga class or a project that demands creativity, or simply to replace their daily SSRI with something "more natural." In Colorado, a company called Moms On Mushrooms, run by two suburban women, offers "education and support, exclusively for mothers, through multiple offerings centered around the sacred practice of microdosing mushrooms." For those opposed to the mushrooms' dungy aroma or to having desiccated fungi grit wedged between their teeth, a local dealer in LA offers a menu (sent via the encrypted text-messaging app Signal) of artisanal chocolate bars in such flavors as Cinnamon Toast Crunch, Cookies & Cream, and Cherry Garcia.

Daphna, however, would be taking a "heroic" dose of mushrooms—not a casual dip but a running cannonball into the inner space between her ears. Renowned ethnobotanist and psychonaut Terence McKenna coined the term "heroic dose" (sometimes a "committed dose"), which was said to function like a psychedelic hammer, "flatten[ing] the most resistant ego." Daphna would embark on this journey in the San Francisco Bay Area with a psychedelic guide and clinical nurse who goes by the name Farah. Even though psilocybin has been legalized in Oregon, decriminalized in several American cities, and cited in thousands of publications in the National Library of Medicine, Farah doesn't use her real name because her current vocation is still technically felonious: she supplies and administers a Schedule I narcotic.

Though Farah mostly practices in Northern California, she lives abroad. She doesn't advertise; clients find her by word of mouth and through a network of hip cognoscenti—a sort of underground Goop. She doesn't like to talk on a regular phone line, preferring Signal. Yet, like most health practitioners and any psychedelic guide worth their salt, she requires her patients to fill out a detailed intake form, which plumbs their psychological background, family medical history, and previous drug use.* She also requires a series of phone conversations in advance of a session with her, outlining a patient's intentions for their upcoming "journey."

My wife found Farah because one of her best friends was among those Bay Area cognoscenti and had done a guided MDMA (ecstasy) journey with her. Our friend told us she'd spent the day on Farah's couch exorcising demons from her psyche, including her father's repeated sexual assault of her as a child. She'd thrashed and flailed on the couch, bellowing, "Fuck youuu . . . I claim *me!* Fuck you! I claim *me!!!*" Our friend described it as physical and psychological liberation. It was the kind of experience that allows psychedelic practitioners to boast that a single journey can provide more healing than years of therapy.†

Daphna's experience on mushrooms was far more sedate, though no less meaningful. The evening after her journey, she called to recount to me everything she could remember: There was a path leading into a Mayan pyramid. There to greet her

---

* Those in the world of psychedelics underscore the bitter irony that society has come to call baths of chemicals cooked up in industrial labs "medicine," while naturally grown compounds used as actual medicine for millennia are called "drugs."

† One such study published in *Nature Medicine* in 2021 showed that hallucinogens, particularly MDMA, have "result[ed] in a significant and robust attenuation of PTSD."

was a lion. Through its gaping maw, it beamed the light of the temple. Picking through the mash-up of imagery after her five-hour mushroom journey, Daphna had discovered her purpose in life: building a musical bridge between the adult and child worlds.

The absence of a discernible link between Mayan temples, a geographically miscast lion, and children's music is ultimately irrelevant. What matters is that the experience was a beacon for Daphna. In the years since, she has accomplished everything foretold by the lion in the temple.[*]

Who doesn't want to "claim" themselves and scream "fuck you" at their internal demons? Who doesn't want to see light-beaming lions that both heal and prophesy the future? I sure did. A bonus was that, with psilocybin, as Farah told my wife, you could go on such a journey without going off antidepressants.

So in light of Daphna's experience, in early 2021 I steered our Volvo north toward the Bay Area. There was an expensive toll on this increasingly trafficked road to Damascus. Mushrooms themselves may be relatively cheap, but a guided tour into the psychedelic realm is not. Farah charged $1,500—unaffordable to all but the well-heeled or the desperate.

---

[*] An anecdote apropos of mushroom trips: In March 2022, after my reporting in Ukraine, a Polish military contractor assigned to drive me from L'viv to Warsaw related his own experience. He had suffered severe PTSD doing contract work in the Horn of Africa and elsewhere. After one particularly gnarly experience, he came home depressed. What cured him? A huge dose of psilocybin. He went to a nearby forest, ate the mushrooms, spent fifteen hours in nature, laughed, cried, soaked in wonderment, and went home a changed man. Well, until the next deployment.

INSIDE HALF DOME

A spring chill intruded from an open window as I sat across from Farah. Her feet were propped up on an ottoman, a notepad on her lap. Around us were rainbowed refractions from a string of crystals hanging from the ceiling. Wind chimes tinkled in the breeze of the San Francisco Bay. Despite our location, Farah's gentle twang betrayed her roots in the Ozarks. She had spent much of her lifetime as a registered nurse specializing in psychiatric care, before pivoting away from conventional medicine. She was businesslike, though her denim-blue eyes broadcasted kindness.

She asked if I had fasted since the night before. I had. She asked about my psychiatric history, not for the first time (we had spoken in the weeks prior). I told her about my family history and about the panic attacks, in more detail this time. I mentioned that I thought panic *might* be the consequence of something more systemic, like buried grief—that deflating balloon Lane had sensed in me—which was why I told her I wanted "the medicine to guide me." But in all honesty I may have been dissembling: I felt somewhat embarrassed coming to Farah as a single-issue patient. Asking her to simply fix my panic attacks was like kneeling at your bedside and praying for God to give you a PlayStation, rather than for world peace or the health of your family.*

Farah asked about my experience with psychedelics to date. Not so great. I described a bad LSD trip at a Grateful Dead concert the summer before eleventh grade, during which my friends turned into ghouls and I suffered cata-

---

* Not knocking nightly prayers. Even though I'm agnostic, for years I'd pray nightly, always asking God to keep my family safe and healthy. You never know.

strophic bathroom stage fright, desperate to pee but unable to. I remained a nervous, self-conscious wreck for the next several hours (and probably a lot longer).

My previous experience with mushrooms came a few years after that Dead concert. One winter in northern Massachusetts, my college friends and I dug our hands into a ziplock bag filled with mushrooms, scooping out what we thought would be the right amount. We walked to a little state park near school, painted white with fresh snow. We were dazzled by the cornflower sky and austere maples. At some point my friends decided they wanted a change of scenery, but I stayed behind to marvel at nature. I walked around for a while, just taking it all in. After a few minutes a new sound joined the crunch of snow under my boots. About twenty yards ahead of me on the trail was a little girl humming as she walked with her mom. She must have been five or six and was bundled up like a mini Michelin Man. She was holding her mother's hand but walking backward facing me. Seeing mother and daughter, hearing those sweet hums, I was warmed by the sensation that all was well with the world. We made eye contact and, with a smile, I tried to beam back to the little creature the warmth I was feeling.

She piped up: "Mommy, that man is scaring me."[*]

Wham! Suddenly all was *not* right with the world. My trip curdled.

It was an invitation to laugh, but Farah, very soberly, took it all in. She was pretty sure this experience would be different. Not only would there be no place to go; there would be nothing to see—I'd have an eye mask on. I wasn't to leave the couch unless it was to go to the bathroom, and to do so Farah

---

[*] Okay, in full disclosure, at the time I had dyed orange hair and a handlebar mustache. So maybe her fear was warranted.

would escort me. She, the psychiatric nurse, would be there throughout, guarding and guiding my journey. This wasn't to be a crash course in psychedelics; this was tripping with an airbag.

Intake complete, Farah told me to stand up. She brought me to a small altar near the door of the apartment and we stood face-to-face. She lit a clutch of sage and traced my body with the smoke, whispering a liturgy of homemade blessings and asking the medicine to guide me. I breathed in the curls of smoke and closed my eyes. As a mostly lapsed Jew, I am a sucker for ritual and all the better if it doesn't require hours of prayer in a house of worship. Farah then instructed me to sit down on the couch and disappeared for a couple of minutes.

She'd gone to her stash, weighed out 3.5 grams of mushrooms, then ceremonially presented the "medicine" to me on a pink crystal dish. Plated there were little piles of honey, homemade chocolate, and the magic mushrooms themselves, like hallucinogenic nouvelle cuisine. Farah called this the "holy trinity" of the shamans of southern Mexico. Alone, the mushrooms taste like tangy dirt. But the honey and the homemade chocolate made for a tasty Eucharist—especially since I was peckish from fasting.

We talked as we waited for the medicine to kick in. She ushered me outside and we sat on a swing overlooking an estuary. I told her more of my story. She told me about her own journey—from conventional psychiatry to the spiritual and unorthodox. Still we waited. We waited a really long time.

With me back on the couch and my eye mask clamped down, Farah played tribal music full of chants and distant drums. My imagination began to welcome slithering snakes, the air-light touch of spiders on my skin, the hoots of half-hidden humans from deep in the jungle. I observed them, but they did not scare me. A feeling of safety can come in several forms. One is the awareness of the absence of danger. Another is the acknowledgment of the presence of danger but being unafraid of it. The latter, it turns out, feels really good.

So far the experience seemed interesting enough but well short of a Terence McKenna ego-flattening. I was certainly observing the world from a different perspective, but the person looking out that window was, disappointingly, still very much me.

I asked Farah if I could have more medicine. She was curious—that was the dose she gave to pretty much everyone. She quizzed me on how I was feeling. The most powerful sensation I felt, I told her, was cold. Perhaps I was getting sick? She explained that psychedelics can mess with your inner thermostat. She asked if I was seeing much.

"Not really. I'm pretty sure I need more," I told her, trying not to sound like a drug fiend.

She gave me another gram and an hour later asked how I was. "Good, but pretty much the same," I said. So she gave me yet *another* gram for a total dose of 5.5 grams.* At last I started to travel.

"Wow, Farah," I chirped, lifting the eye mask from my face so I could look at her, "I didn't expect this feeling . . . of strength." She offered a pleasant "Mmm-hmm." Like a creative writing teacher, she worked to coax details out of me. My semi–dream state (was I officially hallucinating or merely willing my imagination to roam?) then took me inside the belly of a mountain of solid granite. It looked like Yosemite's Half Dome. I was part of the granite's composite but able to gaze outward through the skin of the mountain, feeling immovable and impenetrable. Later I kept seeing the gnarled

---

* As I would later learn—but wish I knew then—people's metabolizing of psychedelics varies widely.

bark of thousand-year-old oaks. The bark was growing in time lapse, as fast as an unfurling sail.

Farah busily jotted down my ramblings. I had expected to uncover deep reservoirs of pain; instead, the medicine was sending me messages of permanence and growth. Soon, though, Farah started guiding me down a different path. She wanted to know about my father. She asked me to go back to that day in late September—the day he died. She had me retrace the fifty-foot walk from the pile of autumn leaves in the street to our door—the doorframe against which my grandfather braced himself to deliver the news.

By now I had turned onto all fours on Farah's couch and was weeping softly. She lay a gentle hand on my back, grounding me and "holding space," as practitioners call it. She then asked me to conjure up my father's presence, and my mother's, to speak to them as if they were right there on the couch with me.

"Uh . . . Farah"—I peeked above the eye mask—"I am not tripping nearly enough to do that." There was still way too much "me" there to reanimate the dead.

After about four hours the medicine wore off. My mind wandered to the rumbling in my belly and my craving for coffee. It had been nearly twenty hours since I'd eaten. I told Farah I wasn't feeling much anymore, and she finally called it. She offered me a sumptuous little platter of fruit and nuts, which I gobbled down.

We got to talking about her work, and how one becomes a psychedelic guide. She told me she was part of a loosely affiliated group of such guides, hundreds of them, who covertly roam the country and world dispensing ancient wisdom and hallucinogens. They were by and large trained by a single married couple who had spent more than thirty years treating and training seekers on psilocybin and MDMA journeys.

This dynamic pair were also psychologists, I was told, trying to preserve ancient traditions of plant healing and combine them with modern therapy.

Enthralled by the notion of an underground movement of psychedelic guides, I would spend over eighteen months learning about them. Along the way, I discovered an increasing number of patients alleging sexual and psychological abuse by their guides while under psychedelic medicine. Psychedelics may very well be the future of psychology (or at least *a* future of psychology); but, like conventional treatment, which is premised on the kind of trusting human relationships that are always ripe for abuse, it requires guardrails, regulations, and oversight. The only way to do that is to bring it out of the shadows. This was something that Oregon did in January 2023, by becoming the first state to legalize psilocybin use in a clinical setting.

But in early 2021 in California, this work was still in the shadows and off the books. As Farah and I hugged goodbye, burrowing deep into each other, it felt like we exchanged something ethereal.

Immediately after came the awkward moment where we actually had to exchange something material: money.

"So, can I Venmo it to you?"

"Sorry, no."

"Ah . . . how about a check?"

Even worse. She said she only accepted cash. I had a few hundred dollars on me (kept in my passport wallet, which I have with me at all times—you never know when you might get deployed). "Okay, there must be an ATM somewhere nearby," I muttered. I bid her farewell for the moment and retreated to my car. It would be wrong to say I was still tripping. Rather, my brain seemed happily in neutral—willing to roll wherever gravity took it. I drove to an ATM, fumbled through two cash withdrawals, and returned to my car with the cash, which I struggled to accurately count. About an hour later, I finally carried a wad I thought was around $1,500 to Farah's door, held it out to her, and asked her to count it for me. She kindly did so and sent me on my way.

I drove off to find a trailhead I'd looked up earlier. The spring grass was euphorically green, the sky so clear I saw stars in daylight. Driving home the following day, I called my wife and Lane and regaled them with the story of Farah and that trip. Lane was so "stoked" for my induction into this new world. Inside, though, I wondered whether anything had really changed. Had that one journey been enough to hit the reset button in the central processor of my brain?

CHAPTER 8

The Dose Makes the Poison

On a typically swampy day in Puerto Maldonado, Peru, the westernmost region of the Amazon, a sticky clump of people, myself included, waited for the security operation at the city's tiny airport to filter us through. The news team with which I'd just spent the previous week slogging through primal rainforest was just feet away at the ticket counters. I was standing sandwiched between dozens of other humans.

And still, I was lonely. I actually had to stifle tears. I tried to laugh at myself: *Oh, here you are, a privileged forty-something man, a seasoned traveler, going to "find yourself," and you want to cry because you're so lonesome.* * *Get a grip!*

It had been an intense week of reporting on the illegal burning, logging, and mining that was ripping up the Amazon. But mostly I was raw from a recurring nightmare I'd been having the previous few nights in the jungle. In those dreams, I kept returning to an abandoned house in the dead of night. Time and weather had cracked and stained its stucco

---

* Note to young travelers: That twinge of loneliness is a good thing. The more scared you are at the outset of a journey, the more accomplished you'll feel when you settle down and enjoy the trip.

walls. As I rounded a corner toward a door, I noticed it was ajar, darkness spilling out of it. Inside I could just make out an old iron bed frame. It was rusty, its paint chipped. As I edged closer to the entrance, the room radiated a stench of terror that knocked me on my ass. I was frozen in place, unable to rise off the ground, but also unable to look away from that darkened foot-wide gap emitting pure fear. In my dream I forced myself to peer deeper into the gap, reflexively letting out a scream-growl. Finally I managed to lift myself off the ground and leave, only to circle back to the door again and again, growling, howling at that stench of terror.

It was November, about six months since my mushroom experience with Farah. My general mood had improved and my panic hadn't resurfaced—I hadn't had a full-blown episode since Phoenix nearly a year earlier. I would get nervous, yes, but not the brain-freezing, underpants-drenching variety of nerves. As the mushroom trip had shown me, and as the series of nightmares in the jungle helped punctuate, there was still a lot of other stuff going on in my head. I had always treated panic as the illness, not a symptom. It now seemed it might just be the most obvious expression of some deeper trauma, a wound demanding attention.

Which goes a long way toward explaining how I found myself in an airport, nearly forty-four years old, blinking back tears. Something was shaking loose inside me.

It wasn't just the dreams. Since mushrooms with Farah, I'd been having nostalgia flashbacks. I would see my beloved grandmother and the little worms of sunscreen that would get caught in the folds of her neck, or my father's impish grin on the tennis court after a trick shot. In my mind's eye, my grandmother appeared in video, my dad mostly in freeze frames. I was hoping, perhaps unreasonably, that where I was going I might reanimate them both—something I had rejected with Farah but now felt ready for.

That fall I had signed up for a weeklong ayahuasca retreat in a place known as the Sacred Valley in Peru. Here's how journalist and explorer of the psychedelic Peter Gorman described the ayahuasca experience: "You take the drug as a small cup of very thick, burnt grapefruit, tobacco-infused concoction . . . The first twenty minutes is waiting, and colours, and lines, and sparkly things happen. . . . That's followed by vomiting, and sometimes diarrhea. . . . That's followed by . . . a dream state, where you really get to see yourself or the world, from a perspective that you've never seen before."

With mushrooms I had nibbled at that dream state, of seeing the world from a life-altering perspective. Ayahuasca sounded like a three-course meal of healing.

I wouldn't know a soul on this journey—and that was by design. If I was hoping for transformation, there could be no social safety nets or security blankets. That meant leaving behind my most trusted security blanket of the past nearly two decades: Paxil. One of the prerequisites of the retreat was being completely clean of antidepressants, benzos, or narcotics. After hearing that I'd been prescribed Paxil for years, the retreat's intake specialist sternly warned me in advance that the alkaloids in the ayahuasca brew could be extremely dangerous when coupled with SSRIs. I assured them I had spent the previous several months weaning myself off antidepressants.

I had begun titrating down in July and August, reducing my daily dose of Paxil by 25 percent every two weeks. A journal entry from August reads, "Everything I think feels wrong." By early September I had stopped taking the pill entirely, and the effect was noticeable. It was like cleaning off the grime from an old painting, its colors suddenly more vibrant. Various hues of emotion now sprang out of me. I teared up uncharacteristically at movies. I snapped at the kids, sniped at my wife. In a journal entry later that month, I noted that this access to emotion "makes me so much more irritable and easily angry and frustrated, and yes sad."

Flash-forward two months. As the little jet took off from Puerto Maldonado, Temple Grandin's words dinged in my head like a seat belt warning: "I recommend *not* going off of it. I repeat, *not* going off it."

When the LATAM jet began its descent between the icy shoulder blades of the Andes' remaining glaciers, I had to will myself to focus on my wonderment rather than my fear.

There was plenty to admire. Cusco is the oldest living city in the Americas. The former capital of the Incas—which Spanish conquerors largely built over using slave labor, installing soaring cathedrals set behind clacking cobblestone streets—it retains the feel of an old-world city, one where people still look different and dress differently than in our modern metropolises. It even smells different, with a scent common to high mountain towns all over the world, a mixture of wood smoke and cheap diesel.

I would be joining a small group of fellow travelers for a seven-day retreat. It would have us sampling a trinity of psychedelics—three sessions on ayahuasca, one session with 5-MeO-DMT, sometimes called "the God molecule," and another on mescaline, a more mild hallucinogen made famous by Aldous Huxley's classic *The Doors of Perception*.

The day before the actual retreat, guests were told to check in at a downtown hotel to get Covid-tested. The group I found when I arrived was older, whiter, and far less New Agey than I had expected. To my surprise, this would be the first ayahuasca experience for all of us. About a dozen of us sat in the hotel courtyard, each person going into an office to get swabbed, the rest shifting around awkwardly in their seats. I did my best to break the ice, lobbing a stupid question, then a joke to lighten the mood.

There were two men who stood out to me right away. One, whom I'll call Brian, seemed obviously ex-military: a dense build covered by sensible outdoorsy duds, a bushy brown beard, Oakley sunglasses. The intensity radiating from his face was almost scary; his eyes seemed to vibrate, a blink away from either tears or ripping somebody's face off. In decades of meeting tormented humans, I had rarely encountered someone who seemed so visibly traumatized.

Then there was the blond stoner kid with the hyper-Waspy name—let's call him Pete. Wrapped in Patagonia, he had a voice fried from a thousand joints. He was obviously the youngest person there. His shoulder-length hair was pin-straight and blond, and when it flopped over his face he would futilely sweep it back with the broad part of his hand. I had him pegged as an uber-privileged kid whose parents had indulged him with this postcollegiate lark of a drug journey in an "interesting" foreign country. When a group of us decided to walk to the open-air market to buy some things for dinner, he asked, puppylike, if he could join. I could tell he was as lonely as I was.

It was among that foraging party that I first became humbled by the members of this group. They starting talking about the pre-retreat *dieta,* an ayahuasca-specific eating regimen that I had evidently ignored in my all my psychic preparation for this jaunt. The dieta forbids the consumption of alcohol, dairy, and most meat (which was why our market purchases comprised mostly fruit and nuts). They also informed me that our information packet had said that sex and masturbation were strongly discouraged in the weeks before ayahuasca. I rarely eat red meat and had read enough to know to abstain from booze the previous week. But I did sheepishly inform them that I'd relieved myself the previous night because I feared going to a retreat like this "carrying surplus sexual energy." Everyone cracked up and asked whether I had read *any* of the encyclopedic notes sent out by the retreat's hosts.

Um, I had not exactly read them fully.

The rest of the group had not only read the notes but had zealously followed their monastic prescriptions.

EVERYBODY HAS SOMETHING

The next morning, our crew of a dozen piled into a minibus for the ninety-minute ride from Cusco to the Sacred Valley. There were periods of silence as the bus meandered past fields waiting for the rains—the Andes were in the midst of another drought—but some of us cautiously began to quiz one another about why we'd traveled thousands of miles for this retreat.

I turned to Brian and asked him about his background. Sure enough, he had been a special-operations medic deployed abroad. Having satisfied my hunch, I sat back smugly. I perked up again, though, when I heard him say to someone else, "I don't think that's why I'm here . . . There was something in my childhood that was traumatic. It's something I'm trying to figure out." I would soon learn how hard he would try and how far he would get.

Pete, the stoner kid, had been quietly sitting in the back of the bus—a cool kids' section of one. Then I heard his bro-y vocal fry: "Yeah, I have some trauma to work on, too."

Okaaay, I thought. *This is going to be good.*

"I was kidnapped in Costa Rica and beat up pretty bad. My little brother was with me."

Whoa, I did not see that one coming. About two years earlier, he told us, his family had been vacationing in Costa Rica when he and his brother decided to go out for a night on the town. Twenty and eighteen years old, the two were walking on a street in the capital of San José when all of a sudden a van pulled up beside them. A door slid open, kidnappers pointed guns at them, and scooped them up. They were taken to what seemed like an abandoned building. Pete and his brother tried to escape but were almost immediately caught. In the subsequent beating, Pete's four front teeth were knocked out. At one point his brother passed out. Finally, the kidnappers, who Pete was later told may have been affiliated with the police, called Pete's father to arrange a ransom. Pete's dad managed to pull some strings with local authorities, and early the next morning the two young men, encrusted in dried blood, were brought back to their hotel.

As the others told their stories, I came to see how all of us in that bus were terrified of some version of that darkened room I had dreamt about in the jungle. We each had a door cracked open to our terror, each of us hoping ayahuasca would help us face it.

SACRED VALLEY

We were driven down a rocky track toward a river at the base of a deep-cut valley. The air was thick with gnats. When the wooden gate opened to the mudbrick compound where we'd be staying for the week, we were ushered through a gauntlet of smiling trinket sellers, then beckoned to join a dance circle. Dancers and musicians with bamboo flutes were wearing traditional Peruvian garb of colorful hand-embroidered skirts and porkpie-style hats. Adidas tracksuits peeked out from beneath the Andean skirts and ponchos.

The lead facilitator, a statuesque Argentinian named Carolina, urged us to take our seats under a gazebo. She seated us in a circle, pulled back her colorful braids, and asked each of us to state our intentions for the retreat. Intentions are a big thing in the psychedelic world. They do double duty, both as guiding lights toward what you want to achieve (rather than just enjoying the trip) and as guardrails, keeping you on track if a trip becomes too intense or frightening. Around the circle we went, guests spending a few minutes saying they wanted the medicine to reveal their life's purpose, help them integrate into their communities, find meaning in life, or deal with the pain of a lost loved one.

When it came time to declare my own intentions, I was reluctant, as with Farah, to cite a single one—like the obvious hope that ayahuasca would at last rid me of panic. That intention felt too specific, too self-involved, too small. Also, Randy Nesse's pronouncement that panic was "perfectly normal" had stuck with me; to have gone to such lengths just to rid myself of it would create a kind of cognitive dissonance within me that I couldn't bring myself to brook.

It was all too muddled to convey to strangers. So, trying to keep it pithy and maybe clinging to a bit of privacy, I offered the boilerplate psychedelic intention: "I just want to go where the medicine takes me." It landed with a thud, smacking of avoidance. After a brief, awkward silence, I was gently informed by another guest that more specific intentions would be better.

The fact was, there *were* things I wanted to experience. Given those nostalgia flashbacks I'd been having, I was hoping to reanimate my father, my memories of him now weathered two-dimensional snapshots. And I hoped to reconnect with my grandmother, whom I had called several times a week in the last decade of her life—speaking to her more than anyone other than my wife and children. As my kids grew, she kept shrinking, but when we hugged, she squeezed with eye-popping strength, letting out an "Ooooh!" of delight. She had died three years before this retreat, but her loss still hurt. It seemed too much to share in that circle of strangers.

Carolina then introduced us to the two shamans who would be leading our ceremonies in the week to come. Reading about shamans, I had envisioned wizened old men or women in traditional garb. These guys were not that. Carlos was a disheveled, middle-aged man with unruly hair and a fleshy face. He grinned often and invariably had a cigarette clamped in his fingers, rolled from the Brazilian mapacho species of tobacco. The other shaman was younger, with a boyish face and a flop of black hair, but he conveyed gravitas. His name was Misael, and he spoke about the medicine with the quiet authority of a person accustomed to commanding attention.

Together they explained how they would run our three ayahuasca ceremonies that week. We were to fast in the hours before the ceremonies, which would begin after dark. Arriving at the temple in the evening, we would wait for the shamans to enter. After some initial blessings we would drink the medicine, sitting quietly until we heard the *icaros*—"magic songs"—which the two men would sing in their indigenous language, Shipibo. They explained that the melodies had been handed down over the generations, but that the lyrics were improvised, appearing to the shamans as they sang.

By the time the icaros began, the ceremony would be in

full swing. The intercom with "Mother Aya" would be open. On the morning after each journey, we'd have an "integration ceremony," in which guests would share their experience with our facilitators and the rest of the group.*

On that first day of our retreat, we were taken to the temple for what you might call a "starter" ceremony. The temple was a long rectangular room in the compound—one of only two indoor common spaces. About the size of a school bus, the room was festooned with Tibetan prayer flags, a tapestry of an eagle-headed goddess, images from Incan and indigenous cultures, and various crystals—the ultimate religious mishmash. We sat cross-legged on small foam mattresses, our backs to the wall. The others seemed remarkably stoical and calm, but I struggled to focus on anything other than the stiffness in my hip flexors and the realization that I needed to stretch more often.

This first initiation would involve *rapé*—a drippy version of mapacho snuff, prepared from tobacco, medicinal herbs, tree bark, seeds, ash, and water.† Shipibo people use it as a kind of smelling salt. It is said to open the airways and the mind.

We lay on our backs as the pesto-like concoction was spooned directly into our nostrils, slipping up into our sinuses and then sometimes down the esophagus. As some gagged and hacked, the shamans explained that they had been given rapé as children when they were naughty—a regional version

---

* Integration, mentioned earlier, is huge in the psychedelic world. It's such a part of the ayahuasca regimen, in particular, that some American therapists have moved to Peru's Sacred Valley, as well as Iquitos in the Amazon, to work with post-ayahuasca patients in need of it.

† It was a dry version of rapé that my kambo practitioner, Brandy, would later shoot up my nostrils.

of washing your mouth out with soap. When, on my third round of the medicine, it got into my eye, I understood the punishment. It burned like pepper spray.

It became quickly evident that nearly everything we would do over the coming days would make us puke, gag, or shit. During rapé and pretty much for the rest of the week, a clear plastic bucket was always placed within reach. We were told that no shame could exist in this setting. It was perhaps one of the benefits of trying these medicines in groups: everyone would become equally disgusting.

The next morning, we were awoken by Carolina with the news that before our ayahuasca ceremony that evening, we would first need to purge, cleansing our systems of various toxins. This part was not in the brochure. Each of us was given a five-liter jug of lemongrass tea to chug, as well as one of those ubiquitous buckets.* We sat on the grass in front of the lodge. Carolina did not set a time limit, but she told us to finish our concoction "as quickly as we could." I summoned the skills honed from binge drinking in college, feeling a stirring of pride for finishing my jug first, and then a twinge of shame for the stupidity of that pride.

Somewhere between two and three liters (about one hundred ounces), your stomach can no longer contain the volume of tea. Most of what we threw up was just what went in: faintly yellow lemongrass tea. Everyone except for "stoner" Pete, who had produced about a pint of evil-looking bile the color of Guinness. It was weird. He couldn't drink the five liters of tea because he couldn't make room for it by purging. He was crawling on his hands and knees on the grass, dry heaving in agony. Beside the twenty-two-year-old was a glass

---

* Don't try this at home. Water intoxication is real and can upset the balance of electrolytes in your system. It can even be fatal.

containing the bridge with his four false front teeth. I realized just how brave this kid was. Now, I was really rooting for him.

FIRST TIMERS

Ayahuasca is a brew made of two or more plants indigenous to the Amazon. The leaves and the vines are mashed up, then brewed for hours. The length of cooking, the derivation, and the quantity of the plants can significantly affect the potency of the medicine. Most commonly used is *Psychotria viridis,* a shrub that contains the chemical compound DMT—a powerful psychedelic. But because the body's digestive track breaks down DMT before it can deliver its full psychedelic punch, a second component, often *Banisteriopsis caapi,* is necessary. Banisteriopsis is a vine packed with alkaloids like harmine that help the DMT become orally active. It is also the part that makes people sick to their stomach.

On the second night of the retreat, the night of our first ayahuasca ceremony, the shamans came in wearing ornately embroidered vestments. They went from mat to mat blessing each of us. Then they turned off the lights. The temple was lit only by the glow of space heaters on either end to ward off the Andean chill. They asked us each to come to the center of the room and kneel before Carlos or Misael to receive the medicine, which was poured from a large glass jug into a shot glass, and from there (because of Covid) into disposable paper cups. Presenting the little cup, Shaman Misael blew mapacho smoke over my head and blessed me, then nodded for me to drink. I took it down in two small gulps. Ayahuasca is called a tea or brew, but this had the consistency of river mud. Its bitterness instantly wiped my mouth of saliva.

We sat on our mats in silence for about half an hour. Then the shamans' icaros began. Misael, the younger, cleaner-cut shaman, sang in a dislocated falsetto that seemed extraterrestrial. His voice was impossibly high and perfectly pitched. My head reflexively bobbed to his near-rapping of the improvised words. The pace of his singing picked up. It seemed as though he never took a breath—singing through the inhale. The two shamans took turns unwinding these ancient songs, said to embody the spirits of plants and ancestors. I was entranced by the ancient-sounding ballads, saddened each time they stopped. The two sang for hours, their solos sometimes entwining in loose duets. At one point Misael took out his guitar, playing in absolute pitch dark, while Carlos smoked. They, too, took ayahuasca during ceremonies.

Many of Peru's shamans are Shipibo, an Amazonian tribe whose traditions consider tobacco to be a "master plant." This explains the shocking amount of mapacho smoke in our ceremonies—enough to nauseate even the most inveterate smoker.

The icaros were soon punctuated by the sound of retching. It was kind of like that famous scene from Mel Brooks's *Blazing Saddles* where all the bad cowboys are sitting around a campfire scraping baked beans from tin plates. Gentle harmonica music plays as, one after the other, each of the bad guys lifts a leg or rises from his seat to fart, soon building into a crescendo of flatulence. Except here it was with vomiting. It's a strange thing that you can recognize people by the sound of their retching. Facilitators darted from mat to mat swapping out buckets. Then came the rush-hour foot traffic to the toilet. I could hear the groaning even from my spot on the far side of the temple.*

I heard a sound from three mats over. It was Brian, the

---

* Sorry, I know this is a lot.

military vet whom I'd been worried about. He was laughing—a lot. Here is how Brian later described one of his experiences: "The ayahuasca let me in completely, she turned me into a plant, I died and returned from a seed pod of pure energy. I could feel the shamans, I navigated the space home, poured love into my son as he slept. Had intergalactic soul sex with my wife, became God. Felt the pain of all of humanity. My hands emitted energy that I could manipulate at will. That's about half of it."

Not bad.

Unaware in the moment that my tripmates were having "intergalactic soul sex" and feeling the "pain of all of humanity," I lay there listening to the group groan, giggle, and gasp, not feeling much of anything. I began ruminating over how annoying that was. Beside me, Pete was evidently having his own profound experience, despite his intestinal agony. He later told me that when he felt scared, a "snake woman" appeared, calming and protecting him.

Facilitators asked if anyone wanted a second dose. I was one of only two people to take them up on it. Shortly after gulping down the contents of the paper cup, I vomited. It felt so freeing to get it out. I was now *inside* the music, marveling at the shamans' endurance. Still, it was unclear whether the faint sensations I was feeling were from the DMT or just the effects of fatigue and altitude. Maybe even just the singing?

Every thirty minutes or so one of the facilitators asked if everybody was okay. "Are you back from Jupiter?" Carolina liked to ask. Most were contentedly off in space. I was planted on terra firma.

About five hours after it began, the shamans asked us to come to the front of our mats and announced softly that the ceremony was being closed. Fruit and tea were brought in.

One man had had such catastrophic diarrhea that he had to be helped back to his room. He barely left it for the rest of the retreat.

The next morning, a fellow guest and I talked over eggs and herbal tea (coffee was not in the dieta). During the retreat I had nicknamed him Kirk, for the *Star Trek* captain, who boldly went where no man had gone before. He told me that, during the ceremony, little alien creatures took him on a cosmic tour of the history of human civilization, from early caveman times to today. During the next ceremony, his first wife, who by then had been dead for over a decade, would take him to see God. God boomed at Kirk to ask him any question he wanted. Kirk was so awed he couldn't think of a single one. He made a mental note to come up with some good God-questions for next time.

Kirk was an engineer by training, and retiring by disposition. He had spent years as a contractor for the military and to me seemed like the last person you would expect at a hippie-dippie retreat where facilitators talked about witches and spirits and talking plants. But the experiences and his time with the group began chipping away at his armor. That morning he revealed to me the story of his first wife, which started, mundanely, with a traffic ticket in a small town on the East Coast and ended in a cascade of horror.

When Kirk's wife—then young and with no criminal history—arrived in court to settle her traffic ticket, a bailiff smelled alcohol on her breath. He had her breathalyzed and booked her for DUI. No one, not even Kirk, seemed to know she was a closet alcoholic, apparently fooling even the intake specialists at the jail tasked with detecting those things. She made it through the weekend without incident. But on Monday morning, just before her court hearing, sheriff's deputies found her dead in her cell. The cause: apparent complications from alcohol withdrawal.

That was a decade before, and Kirk still blamed himself for a million things he might have done differently.

The story was gutting. People came and went during breakfast, but Kirk and I sat there and cried. We hugged. Given how his wife had died, it took massive courage for Kirk to try to find healing through a hallucinogen. Again I was humbled.

Kirk asked why I was there. I told him about my childhood trauma and the self-hatred that my panic produced, and the feeling that something inside me needed healing. It was honest, and yet it felt so small and inconsequential. Both of us knew there was more. It was starting to come out of me, one cry at a time.

TAKE TWO

After the first ayahuasca ceremony, even the faintest whiff of the stuff was enough to trigger immediate nausea in most of us. (Even writing about ayahuasca, more than a year later, makes me queasy.) The night of our second ceremony, the shamans knew enough to start me with a double dose. After the requisite heaving, I lay back and listened to the collective hustle to the bathroom. There was a tremendous amount of commotion that night. A woman in front of me had a severe reaction to the brew and needed to be taken outside for air. It rattled me.

Still, even after my double dose: crickets. I took yet another dose of ayahuasca, with a brief blessing from the shaman. I waited another hour. Still nothing.

By this point I had become frustrated. I, too, wanted to be

held by my mother or greeted by my grandmother, to feel the protection of a giant snake mother, to dance with sequined harlequin gremlins (all real trips recounted to me). But now I was ready to make concessions. I didn't need to see God—a minor deity would do. And while I longed to see beloved family members who had passed, anything that felt remotely spiritual would have been gladly accepted.

Hours in, I crawled on my hands and knees to the facilitator, Carolina, to tell her I still wasn't feeling anything. "Oh, you must be blocked or blocking the medicine," she said, giving me a last little dose. It threw me. *I'm open!* I protested to myself, swallowing the brew. I slunk back to my corner and waited. By now I had taken something like three times the dose the others had.

After the ensuing nausea, I lay back. I felt locked in my body. Behind shut eyes, I noticed a complex latticework of geometric neon designs and a drippy Aladdin-like lantern. I nursed the images like the embers of a just-kindled fire, fearing they would flame out. Okay, I wasn't time-traveling, but at least I wasn't looking at lumpy things on the backside of my eyelids anymore.

By then the facilitators were ready to wrap things up, asking everyone, "Is the medicine wearing off?" Shaman Carlos sang a last icaro, abruptly said, *"Listos,"* and with that we were done. The shamans left, fruit and tea arrived, and the group started chatting.

As we began our informal nightly debrief, I could tell folks were pulling their punches for my benefit. "How did you do, Matt?" they asked with genuine concern. As they talked about God, I told them about the little lamp. "Oh, I am so glad you finally had *some* sort of experience."

Again, I marveled at how quickly the group had gelled,

and that these hitherto strangers had become so compassionate with one another. I worried I was putting a damper on their sharing, and so, with bowels screaming for relief, I retreated to the room I shared with three million gnats. In order to avoid their swarming greeting when I switched on the room's main light, I used the red light of my headlamp.

As soon as I settled on the toilet, I saw her. The glass bulbs of my headlamp cast their red light against the tiled wall of the bathroom, forming what looked like a bust of my grandmother, Mere, the one I had wanted to see. It wasn't a perfect rendering, but it was her. I sat there for a while, taking it in. On the can, I checked my phone and found a series of emails from my cousin. That night she had written family members about spreading my grandmother's ashes in Philadelphia's Schuylkill River.

THIS WILL END IN TEARS

I woke up in the morning starving, my stomach scraped clean. After breakfast, I signed up to do Reiki, or "energy healing." I didn't know much about Reiki, but I understood it involved a practitioner using their hands to radiate energy over the body, to reduce stress or even illness. My skeptical nature resisted pretty much anything in which "universal energy" is transferred from practitioner to patient. But I was trying to be open to new things. At the very least, I thought, it could be a relaxing experience.

The Reiki practitioner at the retreat was an exile from Venezuela named Gloria, who, like millions of Venezuelans, had fled the poverty, corruption, and kleptocracy of her home country. In her late forties with hair dyed black, she was blunt and businesslike. She invited me into the hut where she practiced and told me to strip down and lie on the massage table. I was chilly, but Gloria didn't seem worried about it—perhaps she knew that in a few minutes it wouldn't be an issue.

She began gently by working my hands—*Okay,* I thought, *it's not just energy work; it's fairly physical, too.* That felt pleasant enough. Then she started digging into the tendons on the underside of my right wrist. My eyes popped open to see what the hell she was doing to me. The stabbing pain seemed inconsistent with what her hands were doing. Suddenly, I was no longer chilly but sweating. And then sobbing. I asked her what was happening, and she explained that this part of my right wrist and forearm symbolized one's relationship with one's father.

Oh. This is on the nose, I thought.

She moved to the left arm—the mother. It was equally intense. Okay, this was not the Reiki I had read about. Gloria asked me to turn onto my stomach and began using what felt like a fountain pen to spear the pressure points on my back. I gasped in agony. *Jesus,* I thought, *am I bleeding?* She ordered me to breathe. Instead, I began crying again, my nose leaking snot to the floor through the face hole in the massage table.

What the fuck was happening here?

At hour's end, she asked me to sit up, then held me. No questions, no talking, just her cooing in my ear. *"Es okay, Mateo, todo es perfecto."* I was still sobbing so hard that her boyfriend, another Venezuelan exile, came to make sure everything was all right. He held me, too. They didn't seem flustered or put off. Apparently, Gloria has this effect on her clients. All this hugging and crying with strangers—it seemed so ludicrous and strange . . . and yet it was wonderful.

THE TOAD

A day later, when Gloria came to me bearing what looked like a beaker-sized crack pipe, I should have known what to expect. Inside was a chemical in powder form called 5-MeO-DMT. It's a short-acting but incredibly potent drug derived from the venom of Sonoran desert toads (hence its nicknames, "toad," as in "smoking the toad," or "the God molecule").* The toads are indigenous to the desert between northern Mexico and Arizona and they spend most of their lives burrowed underground. Their venom is extracted by "tickling" the glands around their neck—some liken it to popping pimples. The venom is dried and then smoked as a vapor.†

There were four of us on the temple floor, lined up head to toe on mats. Gloria would be leading us this time, rather than Carlos and Misael. Dressed in traditional garb, she started at the front of the line, two spots ahead of me. Each person was assigned a facilitator. Mine was a willowy Frenchman named Manuel. (Only later would I learn that we had been assigned guardians because toad venom can cause tachycardia, high blood pressure, convulsions, even respiratory failure. Multiple people have reportedly died during the use of this drug in recent years.)

Beside each of us, Gloria placed a lab flask with a pinch of yellowish powder inside. It had a stopper at the top, a thin rub-

---

* This can be confusing. DMT is the primary psychoactive molecule in ayahuasca. It is different from 5-MeO-DMT, which is derived from the Sonoran toads.

† Conservationists are now warning that Sonoran desert toads might be "milked" out of existence. The milking process is not terribly harmful in itself but can cause significant stress when toads are returned to the wild, which can affect their feeding and reproduction. People interested in taking the drug are now urged to use synthetic forms of it instead.

ber hose running through it. She lit a butane torch beneath the flask, heating up the powder until its smoke filled the beaker. Kneeling beside me, Gloria offered a short prayer, instructed me to take a big breath in, exhale hard, then put my mouth on the rubber straw. Then she commanded: "*Tómalo.*" I inhaled the syrupy smoke, drinking it into my belly.

Halfway through the inhale, a curtain was drawn across my consciousness. I had passed out into bliss. "Fuuuucckkk," I moaned, having never felt a sensation like it. But Gloria nudged me awake to finish the beaker. It's hard to know if I did, because I sank back into that pool of ambient pleasure.

I also had never felt what came next: Everything shut down, every sensory input turned off. There was nothingness, oblivion. It felt like eternity. An instant later I came screaming out into the world. I flopped off the mat and onto the floor thrashing, hyperventilating, howling. I was slippery with sweat. It was like a scene from *The Exorcist.*

Gloria came over and held my face in her hands. "*Mateo,*" she said, with a hint of doubt in her eyes, "*todo es bien, todo es perfecto.*"

But I couldn't stop. The medicine had taken me toward the well of grief inside me. I had vaguely known about this well—an abyss so deep I feared I could free-fall into it and never return. I could see why I had spent so many years avoiding it.

Still, the medicine gave me the courage to dive in. For as wrenching as the experience was, I knew I needed it. My physical presence existed now only to scream my throat raw, to purge that tumor of sorrow.

My mat neighbor, Brian, roused from his race across the universe, hollered: "Matt, please shut the fuck up." On the floor as I raked my hands back and forth over my scalp, the facilitator Manuel propped my head on his lap, making a pillow of the crook of his knee and thigh. There, I balled up into a tight fetal position, my knees pressed to my chin. I became tiny. I felt the Frenchman tent himself over me, sensing that I was protected and safe.

Gloria returned, tilting my head up to take just a sip of water, telling me again, *"Es perfecto, no pasa nada."* Nervous she would fully revive me back from that place, I forced myself to sound as sober and lucid as possible. *"Sí, es perfecto, Gloria, estoy bien."* I'm good.

Immediately I retreated back into my wailing.

I blubbered something to Manuel about "the well of grief," but he just held me. "It's okay, let it go, let it go." Slowly my sense of self began its inexorable return. I heard others in the group start to come out of their own stupors. Brian jackhammered out a "HA-HAA-HAAA" and I began to cackle with him. Like sad clowns, our laughter yo-yoed back into sobs, then laughter again. With Brian still laughing, I got up and jumped on him, burying my face in his beard. The two of us, grown men with children but still wounded children ourselves, weeping together. Then stoner Pete dove into our little pile, growling, "I love you guuys."

FIVE CUPS

Coming off that comically cathartic experience with the toad, I felt primed for our last ayahuasca ceremony. At this point it was clear that I was an ayahuasca outlier, and the facilitators were determined to send me off with a bang. When called up to ingest my medicine that night, I was given a triple dose from the start. The icaros started, beautiful and haunting as ever. About three hours in, I was given a fourth dose, then an hour later, a fifth. I had flooded my system not only with an ungodly amount of the psychoactive elements of ayahuasca, but also the purgative parts. The resultant retching was so violent that I tweaked my temporomandibular joint (the TMJ), which connects the jaw to the skull. It bothered me for about a year afterward.

For all of that, my experience was still muted. In the final hour of the ceremony, unable to tolerate the ripping sensation in my gut, I got up to use the bathroom and noticed the room was suddenly pitched at a sharp incline. After making it up the room's impossibly steep gradient to the bathroom, I stared at my hands, which had begun to glow in bright neon greens, yellows, and pinks. I would have paid more attention to it had the violence in my gut not overwhelmed every other sensation.

Toward the end of the last ceremony of every weeklong retreat, each guest receives a final, personalized serenade of icaros, called an *arkana*. It's supposed to be a transcendent moment, a sort of commencement ceremony. Still in the bathroom, I was listening to the arkanas of my fellow guests when there came a knock on the door: "Matt, are you able to come to your arkana?"

This was awkward.

I dutifully put myself together and stumbled back down the steep gradient to the shamans. I was told to kneel near Carlos, the disheveled shaman. I tried, but the pain was so intense, I pitched forward, resting my head on the mat at Carlos's feet. Aware that I was in agony, he switched to blessings that might cast out any evil spirits. He took a big swig of Florida water, a cologne with a sweet orange scent often used in voodoo and Santeria, and spewed it over my head. He then rubbed some into my neck and shoulders. Then another swig that he spat into my hands, which he had me rub together. The scent was overwhelming.

I crawled back to my mat, by now desperately cold and

sticky with Carlos's Florida water spit. It was so pathetic I had to chuckle at myself.

Minutes later, having pronounced the final ceremony over, the shamans stood up and said goodbye to the group. Before leaving, they came to examine me. I could hear them talking softly above me in Shipibo. I looked up plaintively. In the shamanic version of "take two of these and call me in the morning," they offered some more Florida water and left.

I gamely crawled over to the group at the middle of the temple, where folks were chatting over their fruit and tea. My new friends tried to comfort me with Reiki (the non-touch kind) and massage. After a few minutes I flopped back on my mat. That's when something was knocked loose inside me. Quickly gathering my things, I announced to my friends as jovially as I could muster that I had to leave, because I had just pooped my pants. Everyone laughed and waved good night.

The pain kept me up for hours. I felt half-dead during our morning integration session a couple of hours later. The retreat facilitators convinced me to do the last medicine on the itinerary: San Pedro. It's a form of the hallucinogen mescaline and is said to be as gentle as Mother Aya is rough. True to its promise, for the next twelve hours our group frolicked and played and laughed. It was a perfect antidote to the previous week's misery. But my body couldn't take any more of this kind of healing. I was spent, and ready to go home.

HOME MATTERS

On the flight back to California, my back ached. Food tasted awful, even for airplane food. I was feeling fluish. By the time my flight landed in LA, I was a mess. I tested negative for Covid-19, but it would take nine more days for me to digest food normally. I slept a lot and spent my waking hours reassessing what had happened to me. I lost about ten pounds in that time, subsisting on rice, bananas, and toast.

In the literature, online forums, and psychedelic-friendly circles, no one talks about ayahuasca strikeouts like mine. So during my convalescence I reached out to Dr. Rick Strassman, a professor of psychiatry at the University of New Mexico School of Medicine, godfather of DMT research in the United States, and author of *DMT: The Spirit Molecule.** For many years, psychedelics were called "entheogens," a word meaning "full of the god," aiming to explain the religious or mystical journeys that voyagers experienced after ingesting them. Back then, Strassman told me, there was even a theory that perhaps those who were already "enlightened" might experience DMT differently, because they are already "closer to God."

In the early 1990s, Strassman and his team conducted the world's first randomized, controlled, double-blind study of the effects of DMT on humans. They signed up sixty volunteers who would be injected with the drug. When his team injected a former Buddhist monk with the highest dose of DMT they offered, he seemed to retain most of his faculties; he was able to speak and move around with ease. It seemed to support their "closer to God" theory. The team surmised the monk was impervious to the drug because he was "enlightened."

As Strassman told me this story, I started wondering where this was going. *Wait a second*, I thought to myself. *Is he saying I'm like a Buddhist monk? Enlightened?*

Strassman continued. During the study another volunteer had zero response to DMT. The man popped up his eyeshades and asked Strassman if the syringe had gone in. They checked the vial: emptied. Maybe it had missed a vein and was pool-

* A reminder: DMT, the primary psychoactive ingredient in ayahuasca, is different from 5-MeO-DMT, the psychoactive ingredient in Sonoran toad venom.

ing under his skin? Nope. Waiting for something to happen (this sounded familiar), the patient began asking whether he'd received a placebo. He had not, because there were no placebos. The only answer was that this man was impervious to the drug.

The thing is, Strassman explained, this guy was not a Buddhist monk—he was a bartender. No history of drug use, no mindfulness or meditation practice, nothing that might explain his tolerance for DMT. In short, someone more like me.

Then a third patient had the same experience. Strassman said fifty-seven of his sixty volunteers for that seminal DMT trial had profound psychedelic experiences. Three did not. This dovetailed with what Terence McKenna had once told him: that about 5 percent of people seem to have some sort of natural resistance to certain psychedelics. Maybe I was among those few. Or maybe my prolonged use of antidepressants had affected my brain's ability to react to psychedelics, a possibility raised by both Strassman and Ellen Vora.

It didn't matter. Even though I never did meet Mother Aya, I seemed to be enjoying some psychic benefit from the experience. The retreat was different from what I'd expected, but not disappointing. I felt deeply connected to the people I'd met there, and inspired by their embrace both of each other and of their pursuit of healing. I was immensely grateful for the gifts Reiki and the toad had given me.

In the coming months, I would learn that even the purging itself may have provided healing. Following interviews with two hundred ayahuasca healers and participants, the authors of a 2019 article titled "Purging and the Body in the Therapeutic Use of Ayahuasca" asserted that "purging has been integral to the therapeutic use of ayahuasca across and beyond Amazonia." The researchers explained that ayahuasca seems to speak both to the mind and to the gut, concluding: "Based upon our analysis, we argue that ayahuasca purging should not be dismissed as a drug side effect or irrational belief but reconsidered for its potential therapeutic effects."

In our last group meeting before leaving the Sacred Valley retreat, we had been urged to continue our dieta for at least a couple of weeks. That meant continuing to abstain from alcohol, sex, meat, shellfish, pork, coffee, and tobacco, not to mention other drugs—including antidepressants.

Weeks after I got home from Peru and recovered, I noticed that keeping some (but not all) of the basic tenets of the dieta was easy. It came with a bigger realization: that I'd been off my antidepressants for over five months. The irascibility and edginess I'd felt back in August were (mostly) gone. What's more, the panics had stayed away. By then, it had been a year since that episode in Phoenix.

Still, I found myself thinking often about the abyss of grief I seemed to have cracked open in Peru. Was it crazy—or greedy—to think that a full-on, ego-killing, mystical experience might help me not only crush my panic but come to terms with all that sorrow for good?

CHAPTER 9

"I Want You to Die Tonight"

Early in the pandemic, during a session of mindless scrolling, my thumb froze midswipe. A company had targeted me with an ad offering to send the psychedelic ketamine, in lozenge form, to my front door. Maybe you have also seen the ads or an article during a late-night doomscroll from companies like Mindbloom or My Ketamine Home promoting their allegedly depression- and anxiety-defeating lozenges. I immediately started making calls asking whether I was understanding it right: Could psychedelics now arrive legally in your mailbox?

Yes. The pandemic had loosened regulations on prescription drugs, making remote diagnosis of mental illness and remote prescriptions possible. While psilocybin mushrooms and LSD are listed as Schedule I drugs, along with marijuana, cocaine, and heroin, ketamine is listed as a Schedule III drug—the same classification as anabolic steroids and certain diet pills. In high school, ketamine was considered a party drug, one whose original use was said to be as a cat tranquilizer (or horse tranquilizer, depending on where you're from). In those days, kids warned each other about the dreaded

"K-hole," a pit of despair into which one could fall if they ingested too much of the drug.

The medical profession has a different perspective on it than that of my fellow Jersey teenage meatheads. Ketamine is likely the most commonly administered anesthetic in the world. It's used in all kinds of surgeries. It's particularly favored among pediatric anesthetists because it is fast acting and inexpensive and has a half-life of thirty minutes or so. It was the sedative of choice during the rescue of the twelve Thai soccer players and their coach trapped miles deep in a cave in Thailand in 2018. It was decided that the boys and the coach would be fully knocked out on ketamine to prevent them from panicking during the extraction, when rescue divers swam them out of the cave in scuba gear. The added bonus is that ketamine can also cause amnesia. Indeed, when I interviewed some of those boys months later, they said they remembered nothing.*

Closer to home, in clinics around the United States, ketamine was now being administered intravenously to willing adults in cushy loungers—people trapped not in a cave but in the grip of depression. There's even a nasal spray version, Spravato, approved by the FDA in 2019 for treatment-resistant depression. It was co-invented by Dr. Dennis Charney, dean of the Icahn School of Medicine at Mount Sinai, who has been investigating ketamine's effect on treatment-resistant depression since the late 1990s.

Charney says that at moderate, sub-psychedelic doses, offered at clinics and through his nose spray, patients given ketamine might experience a hypnotic state, pain reduction, and an altered perception of light and sound. Some might not notice any immediate change at all. But when treatment is

---

* Which is why it's also so dangerous. It can be used as a date-rape drug.

over and patients are sent home (as long as they don't drive themselves), Charney's studies have shown, ketamine alone can improve the mental states of those with depression. No therapy, no integration, no psychedelic experience necessary.

If treating me for panic attacks or anxiety, Charney explained, he would prescribe three of those sub-psychedelic sessions a week to start out. After a few weeks or even months of treatment, depending on how I was doing, he would then begin to wean me to once a week, and then once a month or so.

That sounded like a lot of ketamine to me. It also felt like it would mean swapping one chemical dependence (Paxil) for another. Many in the psychedelic world dismiss any drug produced in a lab, rather than "in nature," and liken pharmacology—even vaccines—to poison. They wrinkle their noses at a concoction delivered in a clinic, with an IV—while a patient is bathed in elevator music, no less! There's also the passivity of the patient in these clinics: a drug is dripped into their vascular system to do its work unseen, a treatment in which the patient's sole role is to lie down and absorb a chemical.

By this point, having spent time at the feet of Peruvian shamans and sage-waving psychedelic guides to profound if sometimes discomfiting effect, I was inclined to share their view.

RETREAT

For years I imagined my panic as a cancer, which unless completely eradicated could regroup within me. Ayahuasca had seemingly raked me clean, reducing the signs and symptoms of panic. I felt like I was in remission. But I did not feel "cured." I still fantasized about a thunderbolt of a psychedelic journey tripping a full system reboot of my brain. In Peru, I had wrenched my soul and my guts enough to know that such experimentation came at a cost. Yet it seemed now that I had come too far in my journey not to try.

Proponents of psychedelics say that journeys can yield ego death, followed by spiritual rebirth. In the weeks after coming back from Peru, I mentioned my experience of near-oblivion on toad (and near-strikeout with ayahuasca) to my brother-in-law. He urged me to speak to Dr. Dan Gil, one of his closest friends and a psychologist with a thriving multi-therapist practice in LA. Over the last couple of years Gil had been incorporating ketamine into his work.

I had met Gil a couple of times before. He was short-ish, with graying hair that he kept cropped close, about the length of his seven-day beard. With his glasses and low-key demeanor, he could pass for an off-duty rabbi. He projected enough seriousness and compassion that I felt I'd be in safe hands if I took the ketamine plunge.

Gil and I spent a couple of hours talking on the phone. He had once been an entrepreneur before deciding midcareer that he wanted to pursue something more meaningful. So in his late thirties he went back to school, earning a PhD in psychology. Now he spent his days amid patients' sorrow and fears. Even on the phone, he spoke as if in session.

After years of being on both ends of talk therapy, Gil had come to believe that the most fertile ground for healing was a fully psychedelic ketamine experience—dosing patients somewhere between the modest sensation promised by the Instagram ads for lozenges and the unconsciousness induced in the kids hauled out of that Thai cave. He favored doses strong enough to cleave a patient from reality and produce mild paralysis, as well as lots of visions. In effect his goal was to insert his patients straight *into* the K-hole of high school urban legends. It was the ketamine equivalent of McKenna's "heroic dose."

"The medication alone does what it needs to do biochemically," Gil told me, "whether it's through repeated lower-dose sessions or fewer higher-dose sessions. But regardless, accessing deep psychedelic experiences maximizes the psychotherapeutic integration"—or, in other words, healing.

It just so happened that Gil would be holding a retreat in nearby Ojai, California, in a few weeks' time. He could make room for me. The key, he said, was sandwiching the medicine between talk therapy sessions. The pre-ketamine session would focus on a patient's intentions and fitness for the trip: heart trouble, serious history of drug use, psychosis, or schizophrenia were typically disqualifying. Post-ketamine therapy sessions would take place "preferably in that 'golden window' of twenty-four to forty-eight hours after medication."

The more Gil and I talked, the more intrigued I became. Ketamine held some obvious advantages. For one, it was completely legal and didn't require a trip to South America or the subterfuge of communicating in encrypted messages. Its benefits seemed even more supported in science than the previous drugs/medicines I'd sampled. Plus, Gil had undergone treatments himself, finding profound healing.

He told me he worked with a Colorado psychiatrist named Mark Braunstein, who had been administering ketamine all over the country for years, and who would be the presiding doctor on this upcoming retreat.

"He's . . . interesting," said Gil, arching an eyebrow. "I think you'll like him."

SET AND SETTING

In the 1950s, when psychiatrists began experimenting with psychedelics, they realized that the "set and setting" of a trip were critical to its therapeutic success. Your frame of mind and your environment were as important as anything injected into you. In our conversations, Gil spoke of his obsession with curating the perfect experience for his patients. This is one reason many guides of the psychedelic find the idea of ketamine drips administered in doctors' offices so repugnant. Gil had scoured the web for the most noise-canceling of headphones, the softest and darkest sleep masks, the best ketamine-specific Spotify playlist. (To my surprise, I learned there are hundreds of such playlists.)

Then there was the location of the treatment itself: the luxurious Ojai Valley Inn, about seventy miles from my home.

I arrived at the hotel late on a Thursday. Since there were no cars permitted on campus, golf carts ferried guests around the grounds to rooms appointed to intimidating perfection. I chose to walk to my room, finding placards everywhere proudly informing guests that the place had been designed in the 1920s to look like a colonial Spanish village, resting at the foot of the Los Padres National Forest mountains. The hotel was enveloped in an emerald golf course anchored by a four-hundred-year-old oak. Paths meandered to lounges on the fringes of putting greens, where people swished rosé and watched the mountains turn heavenly during the sunset "pink hour."* There were stands of citrus trees exploding with kumquats, lemons, and navel oranges.

Once inside my room, I assessed the ceramic coffee cups

---

* As I later confirmed, the mountains at sunset really do look pink.

from England and nibbled on chocolates handcrafted in Belgium. I didn't check the sheets, but I trust they had a thread count of a million.

Gil's idea was to offer patients the softest landing possible.* If my mushroom journey with Farah nine months earlier was tripping with an airbag, this was going to be more like voyaging in a velvet cocoon. I had to admit, especially after the gnats and gut-thrashing in Peru, I didn't mind it.

Also unlike Peru, where we ate, integrated, and took medicine communally, this retreat was all about privacy. Gil had asked me to arrive the night before the other guests so we could talk alone. After settling in, we passed several pleasant hours in the courtyard by his room, chatting about life, career, and ketamine.

Braunstein, the doctor who would be bringing all the medicine for the retreat, had had to catch a late flight from Denver after his first one had been canceled. By the time he arrived at the hotel, it was pitch-dark. He called Gil to help him navigate the hotel's 220 acres to the compound where the retreat would be held. I joined Gil as he walked out to a little knoll, both of us holding up our phones like human lighthouses to guide Braunstein in.

What looked like a seven-foot-tall ghost zigzagged toward us.† It took me a few seconds to process why the figure I was seeing appeared translucent; Braunstein was wearing a matching white hoodie and sweatpants ensemble, with a diagonal slash of green tie-dye. He loped up to us and swallowed Gil in a hug, his red dreads draped over Gil's shoulder.

---

* This type of experience is prohibitively expensive for most people. An equally profound and equally legal ketamine experience can be had with far less comfort and expense.
† He's not actually seven feet tall, but around six foot four.

So this was Dr. Braunstein. He was about as far as I could imagine from the taciturn psychiatrist I had been seeing in that wood-paneled office in Los Angeles.

Together, we walked to the suites where most the treatments would be conducted. Braunstein kicked off his white sneaks (with metal studs atop the toe box) and stretched out his long frame on a chair. He quizzed me again on my medical history, my experience with psychedelics, and my intentions. I told him about my experience with ayahuasca and my suspicion that I seemed resistant to certain psychedelics. I detailed, again, my long history with panic, and how the fear of panic attacks had hijacked way too much of my mental space for the preceding twenty years.

Braunstein responded with bro-ishly sincere sympathy. "Yeah, man, that's tough. I'm sorry about that."

Gil and Braunstein both assured me that ketamine was kind compared to ayahuasca: if Mother Aya sends you rummaging through the clutter of your past, Lady K offers you a forward-looking journey, an opportunity to write the story of your future. They had in mind for me three intense sessions, which they considered clinically sufficient for what I was seeking. My first session would be that very night.

Braunstein ranged over to the suite's bar for a Nespresso. He would need to be alert. The pair began explaining the particulars of what was in store for me. They told me that ketamine was descended from another anesthetic, PCP. I began shifting uncomfortably in my seat.

"You mean, like, 'angel dust'?" I inquired—the drug that Nancy Reagan and others had warned kids of my generation could turn them into murderous psychopaths.

"Yeah, that one." They assured me that ketamine was PCP's more refined chemical cousin.

We talked for a while before a slightly awkward shift in

which I went from being the ketamine-curious reporter to the patient.

"Are you ready?"

"Sure!" I responded with false confidence.

They ushered me into the suite's bedroom and gestured at the waist-high king-sized bed. I had assumed the treatment would be done on the couch. Instead, Gil and Braunstein basically tucked me in under the duvet. I was a long way from Peru now. There was anonymity lying among a dozen fellow trippers. This, however, was uncomfortably intimate, alone in a big bed being watched by two shrinks.

Braunstein asked again how much I weighed, then lightly muttered to himself, calculating the multiple variables that would affect my dosage: weight, previous experience with ketamine, the depth one wants to go in their journey. He decided to start me off at 1.1 milligrams per kilogram of my weight. So it would be an 80-milligram dose, which they described as a midlevel dose for a psychedelic experience.

As Braunstein rattled off numbers, I felt a silent twinge of anxiety. I hadn't tried ketamine myself, but I did have intimate secondhand knowledge of the so-called K-hole. In 2008, Daphna and I were living in Jerusalem and expecting our first child. On a blistering Saturday morning in July, Daphna's water broke, and for fifty-five hours she tried to deliver our baby. Doctors there tend to believe that a mother should be given every opportunity for a natural birth, but by Monday afternoon our daughter's vitals dipped into the danger zone. All of a sudden emergency doctors rushed in, scooped Daphna up, and rushed her into an operating theater for an emergency C-section.

I was there, holding her hand, as they pulled Libby out. I was told to follow the cart with our baby to the nursery, which meant I wasn't in the room when surgeons began to close up the incision. But as they worked on her abdomen, Daphna started to regain consciousness. The anesthesiologist pumped her with one more infusion of anesthesia.

Three days later it was time to take our little baby home. Yet Daphna was spiraling emotionally, suffering from the combination of a C-section, anesthesia, and the opening shot of postpartum depression. That day, as we carried our little seven-pound jewel out of the maternity ward and into the elevator, my wife recognized the man already inside. It was her anesthesiologist.

"Hey, you were the anesthesiologist at my delivery, right? What the hell did you give me?"

Unruffled, he asked, "Why? What did it feel like?"

"It felt like I died," Daphna said. As the anesthesia ebbed, she had wandered out of deep unconsciousness into a space somewhere between existence and oblivion. "It was the scariest experience of my life," she added.

"It was ketamine," the doctor said. "I'm sorry it was so unpleasant." The doors opened and he stepped out, turning back to say that what she suffered was "unusual."

Daphna's words reverberated in my head as I lay in my immaculate bed. *The scariest experience of my life.* Pulling down my eyeshades and clamping headphones over my ears, I hoped I wouldn't have an "unusual" experience.

With that eye mask, I couldn't see Braunstein return with the syringe, but I felt his hand on my exposed shoulder, pressing down firmly. Over the music I heard him whisper a quick prayer for my journey. Then the pinch of the syringe. I lay there listening to the "Ketamine Initiation" playlist on Spotify and waited for something to happen.

Within a couple of minutes, I exhaled with the contentment of savoring hot cocoa on a snowy night. The sensation intensified until I found myself cursing with mortifying, orgasmic frequency. I know this because, usefully but embarrassingly, I audio-recorded the sessions (with the doctors' consent).

"Oh my fucking god," I declared, followed by a Borat-esque "Wa-wa-wee-waa!"

My pronouncements couldn't match what was going on in my mind. As I descended ever deeper, I began to experience the universe as an infinite flat surface. Like an old-school road map about to be stored in a glove compartment, it began folding itself up. As planes of space accordioned, green, red, and blue oozed outward, congealing into one of those messy art projects kids do with shaving cream. Then all the colors fused into black.

Then there was nothing.

Not even me.

Matt Gutman had ceased to exist. The person who was me had disappeared. So had the pillows, the bed, the room, the state of California, the earth, the known and unknown universe. There was no time, no space, no history, no self. I retained *just* enough baseline consciousness to know that I was a speck in a limitless void, but not enough to know who "I" was, or to recall any prior existence.

You can't reassure yourself that you're just hallucinating when there is no you. It was deeply confusing and utterly terrifying. It was the ego death that psychedelic blogs preach about.

After minutes in that space, I finally mustered the strength to fumble out a few words.

"Am . . . am I alive?"

A disembodied voice responded over the music in my headphones: "Yes."

A few minutes later, I asked, in a little child's voice, "Is this reality?"

The voice boomed: "You are experiencing all of reality at once. This is full reality." The voice was not God. It was Braunstein.

If my experience with the toad had felt like poking my head through the door of "death space," ketamine felt like moving in with furniture. I kept asking different versions of *Am I safe?* Braunstein and Gil called out like sideline coaches: "Keep moving forward, upward—past your anxiety."

My eyeshades became soggy. Tears. I realized I was crying hard. Then I felt a wail form in the basement of my gut, gurgling through my throat. I heard Braunstein through the music in my headphones: "Just let it out, man. Let it out."

I sucked in deep breaths. It was all too much to bear. I managed to call out, "I need to be grounded. Can someone hold my hand?" I sensed the unmistakable meatiness of a man's hand in mine. I didn't know it at the time, but Gil and Braunstein took turns next to me on the bed—it turns out I was clutching not just their hands but hugging their arms to my chest.

And then it all changed. Colors returned, the neon pageant resumed.

Remember as a kid, driving in your parents' car, when you were still learning to read and calling out the words while passing billboards or shopwindows? I was doing the same, only now, instead of words, I was calling out the trippy images whipping past my consciousness: "Hindi music," "helicopters floating across the screen," "blockchain," "pink pigs piling up," "green Koosh balls." (I realized only later that that last one was the sensation of Braunstein's dreads against my face.)

Finally I felt safe and protected again. "Thank you, thank you, thank you, thank you," I muttered.

It bears noting that my experience of ketamine differs from the typical one in at least one major respect: Gil and

Braunstein say most people take the ketamine ride in silence, rarely stirring. They lie down, are injected, and wake to a rubbery mind and body an hour or so later. My recordings were agonizing to listen to later on because I plainly *will not shut up.* At one point Braunstein shouted (so I could hear above the music), "Matt, please stop talking to us. We need you to focus on yourself."

And then I started weeping again. "Poor Daphna," I muttered. It was intolerable for me to think that she had suffered through a hallucinatory experience like this without warning, and without two experienced doctors guiding her through it. She had been utterly and cruelly alone.

This trip had been at once petrifying and, as I kept repeating to Gil and Braunstein, "one of the most profound experiences of my life."

CLIMBING OUT OF THE DEEP

Ketamine had so far been the opposite of ayahuasca for me: all psychedelic and no (bodily) suffering. The lyrics of a particular song on the Spotify playlist spoke to me: "I release control / And surrender to the flow of love / That will heal me." (In the song, midtrip, it seems like it takes an hour for those fourteen words to play out.) It was an admittedly cheesy mantra, but it was effective.

Psychedelics ferry you to the realm of awe, often leading to what in sobriety seem obvious truths: we need love, we need to release control, we need self-forgiveness and tenderness. That the experience presents these truths as mind-blowing epiphanies makes their lessons so much stickier—which may be a secret to their therapeutic success.

"That's why they're called psychedelics," explained Rick Strassman, the DMT expert in New Mexico. "They manifest or disclose what's already more or less conscious. Another term that's new and useful is 'meaning-enhancing' drugs."

Seasoned psychonauts (I am not one) talk about the feeling of being "realer than real." It's shorthand for the sharpness with which we view the world on psychedelics, rendered not in top-of-the-line 8K TV resolution but in 100K resolution with surround sound, motion seats, and Smell-O-Vision thrown in. Braunstein calls it "full reality."

My second journey with the pair was no less profound than the first. I had touched the bottom of the deep end of my consciousness. But I wasn't just looking for psychedelic submersion; I had come to Ojai with a purpose. I still wanted the guru in the molecule to teach me something I couldn't access otherwise—to reveal the secret of life without anxiety, grief, or panic.

"I WANT YOU TO DIE TONIGHT"

On Saturday night, as we prepared for my third and final ketamine treatment, I made my intentions known to Braunstein. This time there was none of the hedging and evasion that I'd offered Farah or the facilitators in Peru. What I wanted, I said, was a message. A mantra, a koan, a *something* that I could bank for the rest of my life and that would calm the troops whenever I sensed a battle brewing inside my mind.

Braunstein cautioned that this was not really "ketamine's thing." "Ketamine gives themes, oneness, connectivity"—he enunciated each syllable of "connectivity" as its own word— "universal truths."

I sighed.

On this night, we would be doing the session in my room rather than in the treatment suite. Braunstein came in and sprawled across a little couch, this time sporting a Rastafarian-themed velour ensemble of reds, greens, and yellows.

"Okay, I want you to die tonight—in your head," he announced. "That is the peak experience with ketamine, when you actually witness your own mortality. And it's wonderful! Everyone who I've ever treated who's experienced that—it was just wonderful."

I wasn't sure I wanted to be more dead than I had already been.

Braunstein decided to try 105 milligrams for this last session. I was the last patient and this was all the medicine that remained. One big dose for the road.

I settled into the bed, bracing for the pinch of the syringe and preparing to "die" (hopefully only in my mind). I felt the jab. My teeth loosened, my voice slowed. I sank ten yards deep into the bed. For all the psychic terror it can inflict, ketamine's initial embrace of your body is addictively blissful.

I soon found myself—or really my avatar—swooping over an Amazonian jungle. After soaring awhile, my avatar landed on a high cliffside, surveying everything below. Suddenly, in what would turn out to be the trip's climactic moment, my avatar decided to swan dive into the rainforest below, hurtling down at terminal velocity. But instead of slamming face-first into the earth, the earth rose up to catch him (and me).

It felt momentous, both in Ketamine World and in the real world. It was an assurance, I felt, that in a leap of faith I would be caught. It was the ultimate psychedelic trust fall.

When I came to, still brined in the drug, I told Braunstein about my experience. "I was deep but not dead," I explained. Still, I had to admit that I felt comforted by the journey, that sense of a safety net rising up to catch me. Could *this* have been the kind of assurance I was hoping for all along?

Still buzzing, I got to talking with Braunstein about his own history. He had battled depression for decades, it turned out. Since he was no stranger to the effects of ketamine, first- and secondhand, I wondered: The healing that he and the medicine promoted, this singular brand of therapy—did it last?

After many years of talking about and enduring depression, "I've become much more in tune with my shit," he told me. "But I still do therapy, and it's still work." He had sampled the full canon of psychedelics, beyond just ketamine. For all the effort, the black dog still trailed him. Almost tiredly, he pointed out that there was no permanent cure to such maladies. "Because life happens. Breakups, divorce, work, bla bla bla. But people can get better. It's all about the work. You don't just get better by taking a pill. Wellness is work." Like most good practitioners, Braunstein admitted he still has much of it to do himself.

With our conversation wrapping up, it was time for his last appointment of the retreat—with the resort's jacuzzi. He urged me to stay in bed. I followed doctor's orders, and since the drug had rendered writing impossible, I dictated as much of the experience as I could into my phone. It was pleasant, taking that buzzed accounting of the dispatches from the outer edge of my consciousness. Hallucinogens barrage you with visual, auditory, and sensory cues: a lifetime's collection of imagery and visions to sift through. If you're lucky, you might hold on to a single image or sensation for the rest of your life.

For me, it would indeed turn out to be the image of the earth faithfully lifting up to meet me as I plummeted toward it. It was a talisman to clutch whenever I feared I might be going off a mental cliff.

The next morning, the darkness of the nocturnal ketamine sessions gave way to the yuppie pastels of brunch time in fashionable Ojai. Gil had invited his guests for a meal before departure. Most made a quick dash for the parking lot, but one couple lingered for small talk. They had done a couple's ketamine retreat with Gil, hoping the medicine would strengthen them as a unit and individually.

Neil and Catrina were showing Gil pictures of a recent dream vacation in Fiji. Crazy thing, I said, but I had just been there, too, covering the earth-rattling volcano off Tonga. They told me they'd heard the boom and felt the shock wave—their whole vacation villa had rattled. We realized that not only had we been in Fiji at the same time, we'd been on the same flight back to LA, sitting just a couple of seats apart. We surely had seen each other. Neil, it turned out, was a well-known TV actor, for whom performance was simultaneously a gift and a curse.

Neil Brown Jr. is a chameleon of sorts. He has played characters who are Black, Latino, and white, gay and straight. Like many of us who appear on-screen, even when he's not acting he's mostly on. We had instant chemistry, possibly lubricated by our ketamine-softened psyches. We were of similar age and disposition, with the same inclination to brace for the bad during the good. Both of us were lovable little shits when we were kids, and both tried to wield our impishness to our advantage as adults. We both struggled with imposter syndrome—never feeling quite good enough. And crowning it all: we had the same tilt toward panic.

The iron-maiden door of panic had first slammed on Neil when he was in his mid-twenties, just as his acting career started to take off. During those bouts, he was certain his heart was failing. Or maybe it was an aneurysm? Cancer? Whatever it was, he was convinced it was lethal. It often came on when he smoked cannabis.

In his first trip to the ER for a panic, Neil, like so many others, was assured that his heart was fine, told nothing more, and sent home. It was on his second trip to the ER that a doctor said, "It's probably a panic attack—do you know what that is?" The symptoms the doctor described made a lot of sense.

Neil soon discovered that that diagnosis—while hardly a given, as we've seen—is just the first step. Not only does being aware of your panic attacks *not* eliminate doomsday fears; it often provokes them.

"I'd be fine for months," Neil recounted, "then I'd feel a bubble pop in my head and I'd think, 'Oh, that's an aneurysm.'" Panic ensued. A doctor in Florida, where his family lived, prescribed Wellbutrin. But just as with me, as for many others, antidepressants didn't do the trick.

It was the unpredictability of the attacks that so terrified Brown—which made him, he says, go "square . . . there was no drinking, no smoking. I was a total L7."* He would do breathing exercises, started going back to church, meditated, tried to "eliminate all stress from my life." For a while, he'd feel good. Bored, but good.

And then: *Wham!*

In 2016, he had already landed the role of the unflinchingly honest Chad in HBO's hit show *Insecure* when he went for a table reading in front of about three dozen fellow actors, the show's producers, and executives. As Neil describes it: "It was a beautiful day, like the first day of spring. People were in good spirits and the executives were excited. We were in this big tent they had set up for us. Everything was perfect . . . and I was about to flip out."

Many millions have watched him on-screen, but there,

---

* A nerd. (I had to look it up.)

with only a few dozen watching—people who respected him as an actor and had already given him the role—he sensed a panic percolating. As he opened his mouth to read his lines, it hit him. "I felt like I wanted to jump out of my skin." Surely, he told me, the producers and execs "would now realize they had hired the wrong guy. I was flipping the fuck out."

Ultimately they learned they had indeed hired the right guy. Chad was a scene-stealing fan favorite. Neil successfully masked that panic. But that same year, for the first time, he started unmasking—first to some of his cast in the war movie *Battle: Los Angeles*. He could no longer hide the stress "in front of the actors I was supposed to be sharing a foxhole with." Then it was the friendly makeup artist on the testosterone-fueled set of the show *SEAL Team*. Finally, in 2020, he started talking about it to a producer, and ultimately to his *SEAL Team* co-stars.

Brown was in a phase that he called "getting answers." There were cardiologists who assured him he was fine, meds from psychiatrists, confiding in friends—all of this so achingly familiar to me. It all helped, but none of it cured his panic.

"Getting answers" also included committing to seeing a therapist—Dr. Gil.

Episodes of panic had waned during his treatment, but they continued to lurk in the shadows. Gil and Neil's wife, Catrina, had urged him to try ketamine. Eventually Neil relented.

Which was how, that late January, nestled with his wife under an Ojai Valley Inn duvet, it came to pass that Braunstein plunged a needle first into Catrina's arm and then Neil's.

That morning, for all our soul-bearing honesty, Neil and I seemed to talk about everything *but* our ketamine experiences. Perhaps those were still too raw and unformed. Those conversations would come in the months ahead, as we took time to assess our panic, the power and limitations of psyche-delics, and what it meant to be mentally healthy. Ketamine wasn't the ending point for either of our stories, but both of us could say that we were starting to feel better as humans—and increasingly free of panic.

CHAPTER 10

The Gold Standard

Squinting at my phone, Michael Telch pronounced, "I just can't see it. I don't see it." We were at a restaurant in Austin and I was standing over his shoulder helping him scrub through a video clip of *World News Tonight*. It was that report from December 2020 about the rollout of the first batch of the Pfizer Covid vaccine, the last time I'd suffered a full-on panic on air (the live shot I was beating myself up about when I met Cat on that Southwest flight).

Telch is the director of the anxiety lab at the University of Texas whose lakeside house I'd visited fifteen months earlier, before embarking on my journey into psychedelics. Specializing in CBT, Telch has studied panic and other anxiety disorders for around forty years. He has 185 publications under his belt and his work has been cited over 10,000 times in papers about anxiety and panic. If ever there was a maven of panic, it was him.

I had sent the video before we met up, and he had texted back to say he'd been unable to find the moment of panic in question. It had felt so cataclysmic when I lived it; I assumed his inability to see it was due to weak cell reception or an issue of a tiny phone screen—maybe I'd even sent him the wrong link. But watching the entire report with him in person, I realized how easy it might be to miss my panic.

In his early seventies, Telch has a prominent brow, below which are eyes that are set back and perpetually full of sympathy. He grew up in Massachusetts, and his father left the family when he was young, leaving little Mike to care for his younger sister and his alcoholic mother. When she would pass out drunk on the couch, her son would tiptoe in to check to see if she was alive.

Then one day, when he was twelve years old, she wasn't. He cradled his mother's head as she bled out from an esophageal hemorrhage caused by chronic alcoholism. She died in his arms.[*]

Mike and his sister moved in with their estranged dad. Telch channeled his childhood trauma into feats of almost masochistic self-discipline. He has held his high school's record for the grueling two-mile run for over fifty years, notching a 9:28 before many runners outside of Oregon had heard of Nike running shoes. Also, decades before the importance of nose breathing became an obsession for some health experts and breathwork specialists, Telch decided to test its efficacy for himself. The teenager drank a swig of Kool-Aid and then ran eighteen miles with the pink stuff in his mouth, proving that feats of endurance were possible without taking a single breath from your mouth. He hasn't lost his sense of discipline. These days, he practices intermittent fasting, eating only between the hours of 7:00 p.m. and 8:30 p.m. The other 22.5 hours, it's coffee and water.

Hard on himself, Telch is patient and gentle with oth-

---

[*] Yes, my father also died when I was twelve. Telch and I debated whose experience was worse, each saying the other's experience was tougher. I stand by my position. Needless to say, it was a debate with no winner.

ers. Shortly after our first meeting in early April 2021, he had sent me home to LA with a voluminous set of questionnaires from his lab. I had dutifully filled out as many as I could, but finally gave up (there were dozens). He'd also urged me to find a local CBT practitioner. Cognitive behavioral therapy relies on psychoeducation—basically telling patients their fears are a "trick of the brain"—and exposing them to their fears. But I had already established that my panic could indeed have catastrophic consequences; plus, no practitioner I spoke to seemed to be able to come up with relevant exposures. So I'd just filed it all away in my mind.

Fast-forward a year and panic seemed to be in the rearview—I was on an eighteen-month panic-less streak. The promise of Telch's "sledgehammer" CBT treatments had stuck with me, though. So, if just in the name of curiosity and completism, I reached out to him again. I had learned enough about myself over the previous two years of psychological and psychedelic experimentation to be open to surprises.

On that second visit to Austin, in late May 2022, I updated him on my adventures in psychedelic land, filled him in on my panic attack support groups, and elaborated further on the way evolutionary science had helped steer me toward self-acceptance. He was intrigued about my progress and wanted to run through those questionnaires together, promising to subject me only to a few of the most relevant ones.

Telch's home office is on the main floor of his condo. Above his desk hangs a scoreboard-sized TV that doubles as his computer monitor. He uploaded questionnaires and we started scrolling through them. At the outset, I told him, "I'm 99.9 percent sure I haven't had a full-on panic attack," with all the accompanying symptoms, since Phoenix in December 2020. I still got nervous, I said, but not the heart-thumping, brain-fogging episodes I once so feared.

Telch reminded me that you can still have severe panic disorder and "not have a panic attack for a decade." That's because, he repeated, arguably the most debilitating component of the disorder is the *fear of* having a panic.

We decided we'd go through the questionnaire twice, first filling it in as if I were standing with him two years earlier, before I'd sought any real help, and the second time answering the questions as I experienced panic now. It wasn't an ideal examination—it was hard to gauge the extent to which my recent experiences might be coloring my impressions of two-years-ago me. But it was a useful experiment, if just for approximating my panic then and now. The survey questions probed for information about the frequency and severity of panic symptoms, anticipatory anxiety, fear of death, and fear of loss of control.

Telch's assessment of two-years-ago me supported what I knew to be true: that for years I had suffered from severe panic disorder.[*] I scored low on fear of death and heart attack, but high on sections dealing with social threat, judgment of peers, and fear of loss of control.

Then we scored my second run-through, reflecting me in that moment. At Telch's long-ago urging, I had jettisoned the magical thinking, breathing regimens, and rituals. I had spent time grieving. I had weaned myself off antidepressants with help from those psychedelics. The second run-through pointed to what Telch described as dramatic change. My symptoms were far milder.

"You went from the severe to the clinically mild range—

---

[*] It should be noted that Telch and a growing number of psychologists and psychiatrists in the field find the *DSM*'s system of classification and pathologizing of various mental health issues archaic. For instance, people's phobias, they say, are often both more fluid and fleeting than the *DSM*'s doctrine—which they think can entrench a sense of permanent illness where none might exist.

which is not completely nothing," said Telch. "I'd be interested to see how you react in the lab."

Telch was referring to the University of Texas lab where he conducts something called a CO_2 challenge. It is one of psychology's favored methods for intentionally inducing a panic attack in patients. It is easy enough to accomplish: just trick a patient into thinking they are suffocating.

LAB WORK

According to the American Psychological Association, cognitive behavioral therapy is an action- and education-focused technique for treating a host of psychological disorders, including depression, anxiety, alcohol and drug use, marital problems, eating disorders, and severe mental illness. The APA reports, "Numerous research studies suggest that CBT leads to significant improvement in functioning and quality of life."

When it comes to panic, Telch puts it more bluntly: "It's one of the few mental health problems we really have sledgehammer treatments for. It can take some years and perseverance. But it works."

His CBT process generally begins with psychoeducation, teaching patients that panic's symptoms are often based on catastrophic misinterpretations of reality and unhelpful thinking patterns, and that those thought patterns can be changed. A practitioner will spotlight those so-called "mental distortions"—*if I get onto a plane, it will drop out of the sky*—and help a patient gain a more rational handle on them. This is the cognitive part of cognitive behavioral therapy. (Though it's worth remembering that critics of CBT say classifying patients' fears as "distortions" is unhelpful and increases patients' devaluation of themselves.)

The behavioral part arms patients with problem-solving skills, aided by gradual exposure exercises. CBT practitioners will, for instance, take bus or train rides with flight-phobics before they progress to actual airplanes. For those with social phobias, Telch will walk into a convenience store and ask the most asinine questions of a cashier, to prove to the patient that no one's really paying attention to most of us. In a restaurant he'll feign insanity, blabbering to himself, to demonstrate that other diners might be mildly concerned but most often are too self-involved to spend much time judging. And if they do judge, so what? There are no real consequences, he says.

There is much homework in CBT, which emphasizes that patients must actively work their way out of their panic or phobia. That often starts with ending the safety behaviors we use as a crutch—our magic underwear or gulping of air. For those with driving phobia, like the people in my support group, ending safety behaviors might mean dumping the cooler full of cold compresses from their car. CBT also calls for jettisoning avoidance behaviors: the ways in which we sidestep situations we find stressful. The work yields not only progress, therapists claim, but a sense of mastery over one's newfound skills—perhaps the most potent weapon against your particular demon.

After completing those questionnaires, I rode with Telch through the late-spring hills of west Austin, across the river, and into the city itself. The UT campus inhabits a sizable chunk of Austin, just north of downtown. It was a Sunday, the week after classes ended; the Seay Building housing the psychology department was deserted.

We sat in Telch's office on the second floor. He pasted adhesive pads onto two of my fingers. Those pads were connected to electrodes, which were wired into a phone. The gizmo measured the electroconductivity of my skin, called the galvanic response—a quantifiable measure of emotional arousal, including anxiety. It's essentially a mini-polygraph. With his machine, Telch determined that my baseline galvanic response was about 3 microsiemens—pretty low. With the electrodes still attached, we walked to his lab rooms down the hall.

The rooms that compose Telch's lab are a kind of torture chamber where patients are gradually and methodically exposed to the very thing they fear most. Terror-inducing instruments include tarantula terrariums for arachnophobes, a lockable coffin-like box for claustrophobics, and, in a cupboard somewhere, plastic replicas of poop and puke for those with contamination OCD. They used to have snakes, too, but Covid lockdowns meant no one would be around to feed the critters, so they had to release them. (*Exactly* where *did they release those snakes?* I wondered.)

Telch then showed me to another room, small and windowless. It was populated by two five-foot-tall gas cylinders standing against a wall—the kind used to fill balloons with helium at kids' parties. One was green, the other red. Beside them was a beat-up leather easy chair. Across from that was an office chair.

The air you're breathing right now is 21 percent oxygen, 78 percent nitrogen, and 1 percent other gases. Carbon dioxide comprises a tiny fraction of our atmosphere, only .04 percent. Breathing high levels of carbon dioxide for a few breaths here and there is physiologically harmless. But the brain doesn't know that. It classifies anything higher than a few percent of CO_2 as asphyxiation. Messing with the chemical composition of our bodies by either reducing or increasing CO_2 is "the ultimate purveyor of death, in terms of sending out alarm bells throughout the nervous system," says neuropsychologist Justin Feinstein, who'd first told me about CO_2

challenges a year earlier. "It captures the entire attention of the nervous system," he'd explained, "and that strong sensation of impending death is why so many panic patients . . . feel they are having a heart attack."

Many labs find that 20 percent CO_2 is enough to induce an attack for those with anxiety or panic disorders. The air in the green tank in Telch's lab contained 35 percent CO_2, a concentration nearly nine hundred times greater than the air you are breathing right now.

In my pursuit of remedies for panic, I had already been introduced to severe *hyper*ventilation through breathwork. Hyperventilation is the presence of too little CO_2 in your bloodstream, producing what's called respiratory *alkalosis*. Your body requires CO_2 to absorb oxygen, and, counterintuitively, all that packing in of air during breathwork only reduces the oxygen in your bloodstream. Your body reacts to this perceived (but temporary) danger by concentrating blood in your core and constricting the blood vessels in your extremities (thus lobster claws and other unusual sensations).

What Telch's subjects experience is *hypo*ventilation. That's when the pH in their bloodstream plummets, producing respiratory *acidosis*. Consuming too much CO_2 dilates blood vessels, but also tricks the mind into thinking it's suffocating. I was about to find out firsthand what that felt like.

Telch had me sit in the easy chair and attached an oxygen mask to a valve on the big green tank. He explained what would come next. He would turn the knob on the big green canister, then I would inhale and hold my breath for a full three seconds, fighting the overwhelming urge to exhale the CO_2.

He showed me a video of this process on his phone—the CO_2 challenge in action. The first subject was a dark-haired college kid with, I was told, low baseline levels of anxiety. He breathed in just a single breath of the gas and exhaled, looking mildly confused. Within a second or two, his face lifted into a smile. He began laughing, letting out a surfer dude's "Woo-hoo." The second subject, a blond male also in his early twenties, had exhibited high levels of anxiety. He breathed in a tentative half breath, then exhaled. Suddenly his face contorted. He looked wild-eyed and frantic. He folded forward to grab Telch, who was administering the challenge. That kid had gone into a full-blown, multisymptom panic.

"Do you want to try one breath or four?" Telch asked. "The one [breath] probably won't be as intense," Telch said suggestively, laying down the gauntlet.

"Okay. Let's go for the intense," I responded.

He seemed pleased by that. Before turning the knob, he had me take several big, full breaths of the air in the room. He then told me to fit the mask over my nose and mouth.

I did as I'd been told, taking in four of the biggest breaths I could muster. The hissing air tasted rusty. Telch then counted me down afterward, saying, "Hold your breath . . . hold your breath!"

That 35 percent CO_2 catapulted me to a different zone. I clenched my eyes shut. Everything went brown and shimmery. I momentarily lost my sense of time and space. "Okay, exhale," he commanded. I whipped off the mask and breathed out. My body contorted—it felt like I'd been fatally poisoned—which is exactly the sensation a CO_2 challenge is meant to induce. I let out an anguished groan.

"Worse than a panic, don't you think?" Telch said enthusiastically as I writhed in the chair.

Yes and no. As I greedily gulped regular room air, the challenge experience certainly seemed more physically uncomfortable than a panic. Most anxiety patients will do anything to avoid the sensation of a panic. Say what you will for my unorthodox methods, but the physical symptoms of a panic attack no longer frightened me. Indeed, even the sensation of suffocation was not enough to trigger a stress response. There was no hyperventilation or racing heart or shaking. Just relief.

Telch had presided over thousands of these challenges. He told me most of his patients just sipped the CO_2, but I had chugged it, which seemed to delight him. "You really went for the gusto on that one—it was great!"

He looked at the app that had been measuring my galvanic response—my body's level of arousal. After those four big gulps of CO_2, my galvanic response went from about 3 microsiemens to 53.6 microsiemens.

"Wow!" exclaimed Telch. "You were extremely reactive . . . Okay, from zero to one hundred, with one hundred being the most physical perturbation you've ever felt, how was that?"

"Ninety-seven," I said, throwing out a number that aligned with the sensation, in that moment, of feeling like I'd chugged cyanide.

"What about the sensation of fear?" he asked. I told him it was definitely frightening. But really there was no hint of panic, or even enough fear to cause me to pull the mask off my face.

For the second challenge, Telch had me take another series of big breaths off the green tank and hold them. Only this time I would be told to stand as soon as I could. The purpose of the challenge was to show patients that, even in the midst of the most severe stress, even in the grip of a panic, our bodies retain their basic capabilities. Think about it, Telch later explained—if panic were as incapacitating as we think, "you'd hear stories all the time of people crashing cars in the throes of a panic." But most people, even those with driving phobias, never actually lose control of their bodies. If that were the case, "people with panic disorder would be prohibited from driving a car or operating machinery. They would be a terrible liability."

With the mask back on, I breathed four chestfuls of CO_2 again, exhaled, and again contorted cartoonishly in the chair. Two seconds later Telch commanded: "Stand!" Which I did. He then shouted, "Now smile!" I began cackling. In a soothing voice he assured me, "See, you're still in control."

He was right. I was. I had filmed the challenges, and watching the video of that second challenge, I saw my limbs were slack, my shoulders low, my head dipped slightly forward. I was the picture of relaxation.

Actually, it was more than that: I felt euphoric. It turns out there's a wonderful release in tricking the body into thinking you're going to die and then not dying. CO_2 challenges offer a unique bonus: carbon dioxide dilates the body's blood vessels, including those in the brain, elevating mood and clarity of thought. It's why Telch says some of his graduate students will ask for a CO_2 challenge before a big exam.

Telch was pleased with the results of the CO_2 challenge but seemed professionally determined to induce a panic in me. He took me to another room, the one with tarantula terrariums. In the corner of the room was that large black coffin I'd spotted earlier. Instead of a lid, it had double doors with a padlock. Telch said we would agree to a time period during which I would be locked in the box in the dark. Not a second more or less. I agreed. After inspecting the box—and finding no "released" snakes or tarantulas inside—I climbed in.

The coffin was padded and had a pillow at its far end. It was not an uncomfortable few minutes. Telch came back at the appointed time, finding me calm. He then took me to another room, this one with a square black box. It looked like one of those large cases roadies keep speakers in, about five feet square. It was filled with plastic balls from a ball pit, forcing all but the shortest patients into a fetal position. When the lid was closed (and locked), there would be no space to move among the balls and zero light.

This was claustrophobia on steroids. It was a Sunday on summer break, and as I lay scrunched in the blackness, I wondered what would happen if Telch all of a sudden lost his mind and decided to abandon me locked in the box in that empty psych department. I'd be there at least through Monday. Maybe until next fall, when some poor graduate student discovered my gamey corpse.[*]

Reader, he came back. And beamed. It was exceedingly difficult for him to induce a panic attack in me, he pronounced. I was starting to feel pretty good about myself and my prospects.

Months later, I described that series of CO_2 challenges to Justin Feinstein, the neuropsychologist. He seemed stunned. "Wow," he said. Most studies use a single breath of CO_2. "What you did, with those four really big breaths, multiple times, that's a very high dose of CO_2. It's a massive amount of exposure . . . and it's a lot of stimulation of your chemoreceptors."

As I was soon to find out, he wasn't exaggerating.

SWEAT SURVEY

Telch likes to work with his patients to develop what he calls an "ace in the hole," a card they can pull when the chips are down and panic is near. Before I left Austin, he wanted me to meet his poster child for the ace in the hole, an Austinite

---

[*] Telch said that speaks of trust issues.

named Jake Becker whose story he thought I would appreciate. Telch invited him over to the condo.

Becker is fifty but looks substantially younger, with swept-back black hair and the now-ubiquitous light beard. Quick to smile and remarkably easy to talk to, he's an engineer by training and an IT specialist by profession. In the late 1990s, Becker had landed a job in Austin with a darling tech company. He was married, living in a hip city with a good job—life was great and looking up. That is, until one Saturday when he had to give a presentation at work.

"And so I was presenting and I just had an out-of-the-blue panic where it just hit me, and it scared the shit out of me," he said. "I was just like: What the fuck is happening to me? I wanted to run away." He somehow finished his talk and made it back to his seat, but he was shell-shocked, lacquered with sweat, and mystified about what had just hit him. The next morning, a Sunday, he had breakfast with his wife. "I was sitting there, and as soon as I put a bite of food into my mouth, I started panicking again. I'm like, what the hell is happening to me?"

That first panic implanted a bug in his brain: What if people notice? What if they recognized his frailty, his failures? These ruminations came to consume his thoughts. The preoccupation only brought on more panic attacks. Pretty soon they were coming in swarms.

Becker continued to work, but the panic became disabling. "I was having ten to twelve panics a day and spikes of anxiety in between," he said. "I was anxious all the time. All day long. Every single day." Desperate, he called his company's employee assistance program hotline. The practitioner on the phone told him that it sounded like anxiety, and that three to five free sessions of treatment should help him resolve it. Since he knew nothing about panic and this was the Stone

Age of the internet, online resources were scant. He took the hotline's word for it, did the therapy, and assumed he would be fine.

But Becker was decidedly not fine. The panic attacks didn't go away.

He started doing his own research. He visited libraries and talked to doctors. One psychologist prescribed special glasses that flashed lights side to side across his vision. The doctor told him to "let it marinate a bit," promising it would work after three sessions. It did not.

Another therapist recommended Xanax. "It was just awesome," Becker said. "But it would last for twenty minutes and then . . . I'd have the biggest panic of my life. And then it became a thing that all I could think about was Xanax. Within a few days I realized this is not working and that it's making me worse, number one, and number two, I'm now becoming a drug addict. Like I'm obsessed with Xanax." He had to wean himself off the drug.

Becker was obsessed with the fear that people would notice his panic. That led to sweating. This was not a shine-on-your-forehead sweat, but the five-mile-run kind. And mind you, this was Texas, with a subtropical humid climate and summer high temperatures averaging over 95 degrees. Becker was under constant threat of being soaked. One psychologist advised him to go to the bathroom to wipe off the perspiration each time he thought others might notice. This led to him leaving lunch a dozen or more times to wipe his face—which itself caused people to worry about him.

Now Becker began to panic not only about presenting PowerPoints to his colleagues, but merely sweating in front of them. He began begging off lunches and hiding in his office—textbook avoidance behavior. This is how people become agoraphobic. Eating became associated with humiliation; he lost his appetite completely. When he did eat, he chose the comfort of the junkiest of junk food.

"Previously if [you and I] had been sitting in this room," he told me, "I'd be thinking the entire time: *Am I sweating? Is he going to notice that I am sweating? It's kinda warm in here, maybe we should go into another room*." But then the other part of his brain would jump in. "No, it's not hot, you don't have to do that, just stay put." It became an internal turf war for Becker's brain, the kind that can transform anxiety into outright agoraphobia and depression. Becker was starting to suffer both. He started having suicidal ideations. "I didn't think I was going to come out of this," he said. When the therapist he was seeing conceded that they weren't making progress together, he suggested Becker meet Telch.

The two immediately gelled. It quickly became clear that Telch operated differently from the other therapists. In the spirit of his exposures, Telch introduced Becker to the herbal extract yohimbine, derived from an African tree bark and used by veterinarians to rouse animals from sedation. Some weightlifters ingest it instead of sniffing smelling salts to amp themselves up. It gives you a weird internal jolt—almost like a sudden, massive caffeine boost. The sensation is uncomfortable, producing rapid heart rate and excessive sweating—Becker's literal nightmare.

In Telch's basement, he would dose Becker up with yohimbine, then make him deliver his presentations, working through the panic attacks and sweats that the herb provoked. After a few treatments, Becker began to notice that, despite the chaos raging inside his head and the sweat pouring from his body, his performance was unaffected. He delivered those talks almost perfectly, then toweled off.

Despite years of these exposures, and of being battered with clinical proof that people couldn't care less about his sweating, Becker was still suffering. So Telch devised one of the most elaborate and creative pieces of psychoeducation I've encountered in the annals of panic. He created a real survey and disseminated it to students in the psychology department at UT—some three hundred people in total. The survey asked respondents to rank the most negative physical and behavioral characteristics from an attached list. It included everything from lying to flatulence, cheating on spouses to differing body shapes and heights. And of course, one of those negative traits was sweating. Out of three hundred people, only a single person listed sweating as their top negative trait.

Becker's response? "Oh my god."

The penny had finally dropped.

On Telch's couch, with the psychologist's eighteen-year-old dog Chloe snoring beside him, Becker shook his head: people couldn't care less about his sweating. "I had this tipping point and all of a sudden was like: 'I am an idiot. This was not true at all.'" It took years of work, but finally—after those torturous sessions with Telch, after seeing the surveys, and after years of his own lived experience—Becker was free of panic. It was only then that, in addition to his full-time IT job, Becker got his master's in counseling. He now works with patients with anxiety disorders.

"Mike saved my life," he told me. Without him, he added, "I don't know what I'd be doing. I would certainly have been miserable." Having heard Becker's story, I could see how well CBT could work, how empowered a patient could be made to control their own panic.

While CBT's psychoeducation and exposures still weren't terribly applicable in my case (I am sure I have company in this regard), learning about the perils of "safety behaviors" and "avoidance behavior" had been immensely helpful to me. Which brought me back to Telch's "ace in the hole." These are tactics that a panic sufferer can draw on in the moment if they find themselves having precisely the kind of attack they've been training themselves to avoid.

The ace that Telch developed with Becker was a one-two punch of humor and candor. It was ultimately what enabled Becker to join his colleagues for lunch again. When he found himself nervous at social functions, he would deploy a version of the line: "Here comes that Becker sweat gene again, watch out." It was such a small thing. Yet it preempted judgment, explained his copious perspiration, and drew good-natured laughter from those around him. But they weren't the target audience; Becker was.

Maybe there was a Becker-sweat-gene-like mental device I could use should panic strike me again at an inopportune moment. For a year and a half, I'd been considering a blunt version of that with Mitch Prinstein. "It would be huge if you admitted on air that you were having a panic," Prinstein had told me—huge both for myself and for the greater social acceptance of panic attacks.

There was a practical hitch to this idea—namely, that it would require the kind of presence of mind that often eludes me during a panic. But Telch wondered whether just the *availability* of such an ace in the hole might obviate my need for it.

I'd consider it, I told him. But I was feeling pretty good about where I was these days. I doubted I'd ever have to roll it out.

THE MURDER HOUSE

I was feeling even better the next day after Telch took me back to the UT psych lab to meet his grad students, who put me through another couple of CO_2 challenges. They were working on a dissertation that would use biofeedback and breath training to teach patients panic mitigation techniques. This time, when the CO_2 challenge was over, my arteries dilated and whooshing with oxygen, a grad student asked about my "anxiety." I couldn't help but laugh. I was just feeling so *good*.

Since I was already there, ABC News had asked me to pick up a story breaking in Austin about a "love-triangle murder." It was grim stuff but also morning-show catnip, and I agreed. As I drove directly to the site of the murder on the other side of town, I was feeling optimistic, even cocky. I had bonded with Telch and Becker and, for the first time, it felt as though I was nearing the end of my long journey into panic.

I met ABC producer Jeff Cook on the street and we surveyed the house and neighborhood—small single-family homes, the kind of place where neighbors still talk to one another over yardwork and where kids' bikes are left strewn on the street. The murder had been committed by a tenant living in a converted garage at the back of a house. As Cook and I were standing there, a teenager crossed our path and walked into the main house. Okay, clearly somebody was home. So we went right up to the door of the owner's house to see if anyone was willing to talk.

I'd been talking to strangers since I learned to speak—to the sometime bemusement of my parents. My grandparents would routinely tote me to their parties, where I'd pepper members of the Greatest Generation with questions about their childhood during the Depression and their experiences during World War II. My sister called me a weirdo. And while curiosity and a sense of empathy for the afflicted have been a boon for my journalistic career, I have to admit that shamelessness has served me well, too. I will knock on any door, make any conversation, find common ground with almost anybody, anywhere. Because early on I learned there is nothing more disarming than just being friendly.

And so, as I'd done many times before, I knocked on the door of the house where someone had just been murdered, ready to roll out my spiel. Through the screen, Cook and I watched a man make his way toward us. We could see he was a perfectly conventional-looking suburban guy. But as the homeowner swung the screen door open, something happened inside me.

As I started explaining our presence on that doorstep, the man's look of impatience made it clear that he already knew. I had intended to ask whether he would show us the apartment out back where the murder had happened, or even just if he could tell us what he knew about the case. Instead, my heart began to thump, my face flushed. I couldn't catch my breath. The leaf blower in my brain revved up and blew away all my words. My pulse went full techno. My mouth opened, but only silence came out. Awkward seconds elapsed this way as I sputtered and then gaped, wild-eyed, at the homeowner, and he at me.

Sonofabitch, this is a panic attack. Full-on, debilitating, and unrelated to any live presentation. *Is this really happening?*

Cook, noticing something was off, picked up the baton and explained to the perplexed man why we were standing there on his doorstep.

The peak of the panic passed in a matter of seconds. After Jeff finished his explanation, I was able to recover enough to chime in and inform the guy (and Cook) that I had just had a panic attack. I managed to chuckle about it, but the man only stared at me blankly—perhaps wondering if all network journalists have panic attacks at the doorsteps of homes where murders have been committed. Cook and I eventually convinced the homeowner to allow his son to show us around. We got most of what we needed to tell the story.

I had suffered hundreds of panics in my life, but they were always triggered by some form of public speaking. Never once, not ever, had I panicked just talking to a single person. I had always considered talking to strangers my superpower.

It was undeniable: an eighteen-month streak of being panic-free had been broken.

I was shaken. Had I somehow been exposed to a personal kryptonite, stripping me of that power? Had everything I had gone through in the previous two years—all the poking and prodding, the puke and tears, the ego dissolution and reconstruction—all been for *nothing*?

CHAPTER 11

The Balanced Breakfast
of Human Experience

I slunk back to my rental car and let the defeat sink in, shaking my head at the cosmic irony of it. My panic-free streak had ended at precisely the moment when I most brimmed with confidence. I had sucked down those CO_2 challenges like a champ, had squished myself in that dark box, had eliminated the safety behaviors holding me back, even had the certification of near-total remission from Michael Telch, Dr. Panic himself.

But talking to a stranger?

Nah, my brain told me. *This you cannot handle.*

After eighteen months of dormancy, panic had reemerged and, cruelly, exposed a vulnerability where I thought I was invulnerable: my joy in talking to people.

For more than two years, I'd been reading about and talking to people who suffered from panic triggered by fears or anxieties that I could grasp, even if I didn't share them. Arachnophobes, emetophobes like Ayla, even people terrified of driving—I could relate to those experiences in one way or another. The one source of panic that seemed most alien to me, though, was basic one-on-one social interaction. I struggled to put myself in the shoes of people who suffered palpitations when a supermarket cashier looked up and said hello.

As I sat in that car, their shoes were on my feet, with laces double-knotted.

I started the engine and merged onto Austin's Martin Luther King Boulevard, then opened the windows and took a breath. Okay, maybe I didn't need to catastrophize this new panic. Maybe it had been a onetime panic-purge, a freak reaction to having thought of nothing *but* panic during the previous several days in Telch's company. Hell, maybe this was a gift, a new pathway to compassion. As a lifelong collector of experience, I thought maybe I should classify that doorstep panic as a collector's item, adding it to the mantel in my mind where I collected stories—mine and others—that helped me better understand the human condition.

By the time I arrived at the hotel, I had reconciled myself with my panic at the murder house. Hey, it had even given me the opportunity to pull out my ace in the hole. It was the first time, in twenty-two years of panic attacks, that I had acknowledged in real time that I was in the throes of one. Just as Telch said, the worst was over in less than a minute. And critically, I regained enough composure to do the work I had been called upon to do.

At dinner that night I shared my history of panics with Jeff Cook. He was sympathetic. By the time we walked back to our hotel to get some sleep ahead of our 3:00 a.m. *Good Morning America* alarm, my mindset had evolved from despair to gratitude.

That said, the mauling by a novel (to me) species of panic did leave me a bit tender. I was still feeling raw during our live shot for *GMA*, and later that morning when the calls started coming in.

The first was from Deputy Bureau Chief Bonnie McLean

again. There was tension in her voice. She explained that there had been a shooting incident in the vicinity of an elementary school near San Antonio, in a town neither of us had ever heard of. Initial reports were all over the place: Was there a single shooter or multiple shooters? Was the elementary school even the target? Why was the border patrol involved? Were they shooting at migrants? McLean asked me to call my contacts in Texas law enforcement.

The more sources I called, the more the fog was lifted, revealing only horror: A gunman had entered an elementary school in the small Texas town of Uvalde, about eighty-five miles west of San Antonio. Children were among the dead. One source told me ABC might want to send multiple teams—I was cautioned there could be as many as ten casualties. A few minutes later: *No, that's not right. It's now fourteen dead children.* Then another call: *Matt, that number is going to rise—probably more than eighteen.* Ultimately nineteen children and two teachers were murdered in the attack at Uvalde, by an eighteen-year-old armed with an AR-style rifle.

Helping my ABC colleagues report out the details of the story would be one thing. Covering the Uvalde horror in person would be another. On any other day it would be a no-brainer (though every reporter will tell you a school shooting is the genre of story they most dread). But fresh off those CO_2 challenges and that bolt-from-the-blue panic, I was a walking exposed nerve. Every fiber of my being screamed out: *Avoid this story.*

I had learned a lesson in the more than two years since my suspension: Sometimes the right answer is no. I told my managers at ABC News that I was sorry, I just couldn't do it. I reminded them that I had suffered PTSD after another San Antonio–area shooting, the Sutherland Springs church massacre, in which twenty-six people were gunned down. It was late

2017 and I had come off back-to-back-to-back assignments, covering the monstrous Hurricane Harvey; then the deadliest shooting in American history, in Las Vegas, in which fifty-eight people were killed; then the fires in Northern California that killed twenty-two and incinerated whole neighborhoods. Over seven weeks of nearly nonstop reporting, I had absorbed a monumental amount of human suffering. In Sutherland Springs, while interviewing a mother whose teenage daughter had been killed, I just lost it—drowning in the cumulative sadness of it all. I apologized to the mother, ashamed that, in the face of her unimaginable trauma, *I* was the one who couldn't keep myself together. I retreated to my car and wept.

Interviewing a bereaved parent requires empathy, and empathy requires vulnerability. On this day five years later, I feared what might happen if I peeled off my emotional armor to interview a survivor or a parent who had lost a child to gun violence. Plus, the Uvalde story was too painfully close to home—these children were basically the same age as my son.

My managers understood. They told me that if I didn't feel up to it, I shouldn't go.

That should have been a relief. Except, I knew the calculus: I was *already* in Texas. If I sat this out, another ABC News team from elsewhere in the country would have to be launched, arriving only the next day. My managers were okay with that, but I knew it would put us behind on a huge story at a time when all of America was clamoring for answers. So after a few difficult conversations with my wife, I informed them I'd changed my mind: I was going.

I grabbed a coffee and headed south on the I-35. Somewhere near San Marcos, Texas, I started sobbing so hard I had to pull off the highway.* My sense of duty to tell people's

---

* Multiple other colleagues told me they had to do the same.

stories was at war with my sense of self-preservation. Right now, self-preservation was winning. I desperately needed to talk to someone. I called Telch, but his phone went to voice-mail. Then I called Becker—Telch's poster child patient who himself had become a therapist. Maybe I secretly hoped he would urge me to take care of myself and let someone else do the story.

His response surprised me. "This is what you do, this is an important story to tell, and you should probably go," he said.

Dammit, I thought. *He's right. This* is *what I do.*

I merged back onto the interstate.

My mind flashed back to January 2020 and the cata-strophic reporting error that set me on my journey to begin with. As then, it was critical that I get to the scene quickly. There would be police barriers to get through, intel to gather, eyewitness and neighbors to interview. In the first hours after such trauma, the memory of witnesses is still fresh—not yet muddled by anything they've heard from neighbors or seen on cable news. Time would be of the essence if I wanted to get the facts and get them right.

As I drove and made calls, manically coordinating the few hours ahead of me, the hallmarks of a panic-inducing live shot were lined up. There was the trauma, the urgency, the feeling of a story all too close to home. I could sense the traf-fic on the highway of my mind beginning to stall. But just as quickly, those agonizing thoughts found their off-ramp.

I got to Uvalde that evening, knocking on the door of every bungalow on the street where the shooter had begun his rampage. Again, shell-shocked homeowners who had been too close to murder came warily to the door, where a stranger awaited to ask them questions. This time, there was no panic. I explained to them who I was and what I was doing. They opened up to me, describing the horror they had seen and revealing what they knew about the shooter, his self-harming, his stalking of friends and death threats to other children. So many warning signs missed.

In the coming days, as we investigated the cascade of failures that led to the deaths of so many children, there would be multiple live special events. I would do lots of live shots in that deeply wounded town. I was able to make room for this new sorrow; I had found ways of emptying my container of grief.

My reporting went without incident. Panic was simply not an issue.

Was I "cured"? Maybe.

Another answer: Maybe that was the wrong question.

THE BULLET TRAIN

In the months after our ketamine sessions in Ojai, I caught up with Neil Brown Jr., the actor who'd been trying to beat back panic for more than a decade. I asked if he wanted to meet for breakfast or lunch. Nah, that wasn't his speed, Neil informed me. Instead, he suggested I come over and work out in his garage, which he calls his "Pain Palace."

He wasn't kidding. His was a professional-grade gym—so crammed with equipment and weights that unless everything is returned to its rightful place his garage door won't close.

Maybe heaving dumbbells wasn't the ideal setting for a searching conversation about the delicate work of managing one's own anxiety. But it's a place that makes sense to Neil, where he can notch lots of small wins. Those little wins build not just the body, he says, but the superstructure of his overall well-being. The Pain Palace also very well encapsulates the dissonance of a muscle-wrapped martial arts black belt who plays a SEAL Team operator on TV but whose greatest talent, in his own estimation, is his ability to cry convincingly on cue.

We got to talking about his ketamine sessions, the subject we had sidestepped months earlier. He said he had endured seven mini-panics during his first treatment. Yet somehow his brain had seemed to work through it. Braunstein and Gil noted that his heart rate had never budged. There were no physical symptoms of panic, only the fear taking place in his mind. He recalled going through doors. Each time, as he felt the revving of his heart and the flutter of panic, a light pulled him to safety. Several times it was his wife, Catrina, who materialized before him in the form of a spectral creature that he described as "pure soul."

Despite a few emotional knuckleballs thrown his way recently, he hadn't suffered a panic since his ketamine treatment, he said. Practitioners say the benefits of ketamine, like most psychedelics, wear off after weeks or months. But Neil, like me, keeps a treasure box of images from those journeys. Opening it up and gazing back on those experiences helps reanimate some of their healing power.

I still think about embodying Yosemite's Half Dome from my time with Farah, and the rising of the jungle to catch me in ketamine world, and the naked catharsis of 5-MeO-DMT on a mat in Peru. I am most easily able to access those images during meditation. This in turn has improved my meditation practice—I'm drawn to that little treasure box, which makes meditation not only beneficial but welcome. So I grab a few minutes here and there—before I get out of bed, during the day, and often when I tuck my son in during bedtime. It calms both of us.

I mentioned this to my friend and former ABC colleague Dan Harris, the author of *10% Happier,* who pointed to numerous studies showing that meditation, when practiced with diligence, can encourage neuroplasticity, reprogramming the brain in a way not dissimilar to psychedelics. If psychedelics are the bullet train to neuroplasticity, meditation takes you there in baby steps. The one isn't a substitute for the other, but they work hand in hand with a harmony I hadn't expected.

Harris is one of the nation's chief apostles of the gospel of meditation. He has spent more than 150 days on silent meditation retreats and many thousands of hours meditating. He says the key to surviving silent meditation retreats (and life) is self-compassion, "which can take the edge off of that perfection [impulse], in a way that, oddly, will make you more perfect. In other words, not trying so hard to be perfect, giving yourself a break, has actually been shown to help you do better at reaching your goals."

It makes sense. After all, finding pathways to empathy with interview subjects, from the victims of murder to their perpetrators, has been my best asset as a journalist. It enables me to connect with nearly everyone. Why shouldn't I apply that more liberally to myself?

Self-compassion is the flip side of the Golden Rule: Do unto yourself as you would have others do unto you. Harris points out that this philosophy is a primary step in the extreme makeover of our inner voice from drill sergeant to coach. For many years, my inner drill sergeant would scream into my mind's bullhorn: *You're blithering! You're not worthy of your peers! You're going to fail!* I'm pleased to say that my drill sergeant has gone into semi-retirement. Also given his pink slip is my psyche's internal statistician—the tyrant who grades my every performance and interaction and who succeeded only in pathologizing my panic. I hope he finds some nice new hobbies.

FREE THERAPY

I'm keenly aware how easy it is to fall off the wellness wagon. As Dr. Mark Braunstein pointed out during our ketamine sessions, "Life happens. Breakups, divorce, work, bla bla bla." It takes constant maintenance to focus on the whole human.

During the trek through my psyche over the past couple of years, I was often reminded of what holistic psychiatrist Ellen Vora called "portals to pain." I had poked my head into those portals, sometimes deliberately and sometimes by surprise. After psychedelics—and the delight, the physical suffering, the ego death they offered—I was now far less afraid of the dark recesses of my mind.

That made it possible to access the "portals" when not under the influence of some exotic plant or animal venom. In 2022, my family took a spring break trip to England, at the end of which I was asked to stay for work. During most of our time together as a family, when I should have been basking in clotted-cream-and-scone sugar highs and watching my kids run amok among the bluebells of the Cotswolds, I was moody.* I couldn't pin down the reason. After the family flew home, I was walking down the hallway of my London hotel when I felt a sadness as physically potent as a wave of nausea.

Instead of burying it, as I had done for decades by, say, lacing up my sneakers and heading out for a run, I swiped myself into my room and torpedoed into the pillows, willing myself to cry. It didn't take much, and once the dam broke it came flooding out of me. I howled and screamed into the pillows until the down got soggy. I lay there weeping with

---

* Lest you think my children are not human, the ratio of them frolicking happily to them swatting mercilessly at each other was probably 1:5.

little inhibition for forty-five minutes, exorcising as much of the pain as I could.

And yes, I'm aware that by now the frequency of these pillow-soaking episodes might make me sound like a basket case. But describing it to Dr. Vora later, it felt less like a cause for concern or shame and more like an achievement. I had first tracked her down after hearing her on an episode of the podcast *Pulling the Thread*. The episode's blurb began with this quote from Vora: "I think we're due for a cultural rebranding around crying."

Amen, declared my internal congregation. I listened to the podcast more than once. When Vora and I spoke, she elaborated on the idea. She sees crying as the body's way of digesting "unmetabolized grief." When I told her I'll probably spend the rest of my life parsing the specific causes of grief, she countered that too much of the routine analysis that some of us undergo with our therapists may miss the "free therapy" of crying.

"Right now, when we start to cry, we apologize," she explained. "We say, 'I'm sorry, I'm sorry.' We suck it back in and try to make it as small as possible." Think about it: Even in therapy [or interviews], what's the first thing a therapist does when you start to cry? They hand you a box of tissues. It's a form of empathy, but also part of our cultural impulse to stifle, mop up, and absorb tears. Vera calls for the opposite. Crying is one of *Homo sapiens'* most efficient forms of release. Look no further than children, even teens, who "are still connected to their body's need for relief. For better or worse, if they need a meltdown, they have a meltdown. It's a train that you cannot stop. But as social adults, we have so many locks in place that can triage our cries, and we can say, 'Okay, not now. It's not a good time, maybe later.'" Too often that later never comes.

These days, I more closely monitor my emotional radar for incoming grief. It's a necessary skill, which I augment by remaining on the lookout for a good, preemptive catharsis, whether from a psychedelic experience (at the right moment, with the right guide) or from breathwork. There's plenty of good science to explain the near-euphoric lightness we feel post-cry. Emotional tears, as opposed to tears meant to flush something out of our eyes, release the feel-good hormones oxytocin and endorphins.

There's another form of free therapy that we often over-look: laughing, particularly at ourselves. I cannot tell you how many times during the reporting for this book that I LOLed to myself about the absurdity of my situation. After all, I was a grown man who owned pairs of "lucky" undies. I also laughed at the ridiculousness of the stories we are told and we tell ourselves, like my mother's *wink-wink* "you could be a prophet" schtick, or the absurdity that anyone really expects or even wants us to be perfect. The crying and the laughter are all part of this often ridiculous human experience.

Evolution is pretty clear that we humans are bound to the same immutable laws of nature as other animals. The well-ness industry's much-flogged primacy of "happiness" is mis-guided, Vora says: "I no longer think the goal is to always be happy, content, and calm. I think the goal is to have a full, complete human experience and to be able to have a through-line to balance. And grief is absolutely part of a balanced breakfast in this human experience." Meaning, not just that grief is natural, but that expressing it, and crying it out of our bodies if necessary, is also natural and desirable. And so joy is something that we achieve, a success we can pat ourselves on the back about.

SO WHAT NOW?

It's hard to measure the absence of something.

I'm three rungs up on a stepladder in front of Van Nuys Middle School in LA. The ladder is an unusual touch, but the middle schoolers trooping by kept flashing middle fingers to the camera, so the crew thought it best to frame me above the barrage of birds.

A few hours earlier, when I got the first call, the story was that ten middle schoolers had overdosed on fentanyl, which sounded horrific and generated instant headlines (and concern: my daughter went to a nearby middle school at the time). But when I got to the scene, I quickly learned that this was not fentanyl. A fire captain told me it seemed the kids had suffered "mild to moderate symptoms" from . . . marijuana.

The fact that some kids got super-stoned on a bad batch of pot brownies was decidedly *not* national news. But on a slowish news day in the late fall of 2022, it was enough to cross a low bar. My crew and I were told to stay the course and prepare for a live shot. I drove home, dashed off a script, and took the 101 back to Van Nuys. Traffic was light and I got back to the school with time to kill. I talked to the school cop about his stoned wards. He shook his head in weary resignation.

Now I'm with my crew, one of my favorites. The soundman begins to tell us about his inbred Saint Bernard siblings. Unbeknownst to him, the brother and sister mated one day and he awoke to a surprise litter of even *more deeply* inbred puppies. We sputter and laugh in disgust.

The weather is damp and cool. My body feels . . . normal.

David Muir tosses to our prerecorded report, and soon the director is in my ear:

"Forty-five seconds to your tag, Matt."

Standing on my perch, camera and lights trained on me, it dawns on me that all the old ingredients of a typical panic are in place: a near-zero-stakes story on a forgettable news day, a stationary live shot, a short tag. There's no possible reason not to ace this. I acknowledge the thought and then gently file it away.

"Thirty seconds."

I take the measure of my day's caffeine intake. A lot? A little? Not sure. It doesn't matter all that much.

"Fifteen seconds."

The cars on my train of thought are clacking ahead toward the tag—a tidbit about the investigation, coupled with an admonishment from officials to parents about the danger of narcotics that might come disguised as everyday lollipops, gummy bears, and chocolates.

"Ten."

A little bump of adrenaline. It's not panic. And if it was, I'd deal with it. Having bared so much by now, I have little left to hide.

"Gutman, coming to you in five, four, three . . ."

Afterword

E arly on in this journey, toward the beginning of my first mushroom experience with Farah, I had asked her: "What works?" With sage smoke still thick in the air, she offered the answer a shaman in southern Mexico had once told her: "Everything."

Reading this book, you've seen that *everything*, or almost everything, is what I tried. Everything worked, some things more than others. I can safely tell you that there is no "right medicine." But there is good medicine.

I'd love to say that, through my years of study, self-experimentation, and soul-searching, I've got it all figured out now, and here's *the* address to plug into your Waze app to navigate your way out of panic. It's not that easy. What I can tell you with certainty is that no one has all the answers. There are, however, a bunch of helpful tips and best practices (good medicine) that I've pocketed along the way and that have gotten me through panic and anxiety. I hope they can be useful to you as well.

1. Knowledge. Remember that a panic attack is fleeting. The worst of it is the period of the body's assessment of danger. That lasts for fifteen seconds to a minute. Know that you *can* get through those first terrifying seconds. It will not kill you. I promise. After that, it's "just" anxiety you're feeling. Anxiety is something you've handled your whole life. You've got this. Also remember that panic is not nearly as incapacitating as you think. If it were, people with panic disorder would be crashing cars all the time and prohibited from driving. That's not the case.

2. **There is help out there.** If you think you need it, you do. The Anxiety and Depression Association of America and the National Alliance on Mental Illness have some additional resources and information.

3. **Don't let it fester.** Let it out into the open. Talk to someone you trust. It can be anyone. Even if disclosure doesn't cure you of your panic, it can heal other things that are hurt. If you feel like you might overburden friends or family, try to find a therapist. If you can't afford one, try the clergy, a chaplain, or a rabbi—they can be helpful (and are free). Also, those of you who have faith: lean on it. It works.

4. **Breathe.** The way you breathe changes the chemistry of your blood. Breathe too fast and you'll deprive your body of the carbon dioxide it needs to get oxygen into your system. So slow it down. Practice inhalations and exhalations through your nose. And yes, try breathwork. There are plenty of excellent classes you can pick up on YouTube, so you can huff and puff from the comfort of your home.

5. **Cry.** Especially you reluctant men out there. As Dr. Ellen Vora says, it's free therapy, and the body's natural way

of sloughing off anxiety and grief. It's temporary, but I promise you, the harder you cry, the better you will feel afterward. The relief is chemical, and it lasts a good while.

6. Move. Do yoga, bench press, breathwork, Jazzercise, Twister, walk the dog for an extra five minutes, take the stairs at the parking garage—anything that gets you moving. When you are exercising, you are drugging yourself. You probably know that the post-exercise feel-good hormones are called endorphins. But did you know that the word *endorphins* is short for "endogenous morphine"? In other words, it's morphine produced naturally in your body—one of the reasons you feel so good after even a ten-minute walk. It's the healthiest indulgence. If you can't do any of the above, that's okay, too! But remember that any added step you take in your day, any minute spent standing or stretching or doing a single air squat, is a win. Don't get sucked into the tyranny of perfection.

7. Meditate. It's not the bullet train to neuroplasticity, but it works. Even a few minutes here or there can help. Again, it's as much about notching little wins as it is about getting to some unreachable place of Zen.

8. Cognitive behavioral therapy. It's the therapy gold standard. CBT doesn't work for everyone, and critics say it can invalidate people's fears. That said, it *has* worked for millions. Try it. Also feel free to cherry-pick elements of CBT that might work for you, as I did. One thing CBT and Michael Telch proved to me early on was that my safety behaviors only compounded the intensity of my panics. Eliminating some or all of your safety behaviors could go a long way in reducing the intensity and frequency of your panics.

9. Pharmacology. Yeah, I know. I made a big deal of SSRIs and benzos not helping my panic. That's true. It's also true that the right meds, prescribed by a trusted psychiatrist, can work wonders for some. No one should suffer unnecessarily, and not everyone has the time or resources for CBT or the other treatments I've noted. Also, most SSRIs are now generic and cheap. But keep in mind that they can be addictive and can cause withdrawal symptoms when you go off them (and possibly also when you don't, as with Elaine Vora's point about interdose withdrawal). If you try benzos, remember they can be especially addictive.

10. Ketamine. I say this with caution, because while research has begun to demonstrate its efficacy—certainly in the shorter term—ketamine may have health consequences we don't yet know. That said, it is, to date, the most accessible hallucinogen, both literally and psychedelically. It's legal and probably being infused in a clinic near you. It's not always cheap, but it could be worth it.

11. Mushrooms or MDMA. The gentler gates into the psychedelic world. If you choose this route, please do so with caution and use a guide. Vet your guide; consult with others who have worked with them. Do a bit of googling. Do not go blindly into the world of psychedelics.

12. Ayahuasca. Not for everyone (see Chapter 8) but life-changing for some (see Chapter 8).

13. Hypnosis. Barely mentioned in these pages, but I've tried it a few times and it worked for some things. (And yes, I had a big cathartic cry under hypnosis.)

I cannot tell you what to do with your body. I will, however, plead with you to be kind. To others, to your body, and especially to yourself. Trust me, I pummeled myself for years. Self-bashing—even if it feels honest in the moment—won't get you anywhere. Remember the famous couplet from the poet Rainer Maria Rilke: "Let everything happen to you: beauty and terror. Just keep going. No feeling is final."

Acknowledgments

I wrote my first book in about a month—a frantic endeavor to meet my publisher's deadline. This book was more than three years in the making. Writing about the deeply personal is difficult. Every anecdote, every self-referential comment is scrutinized by a writer's harshest critic, i.e., himself (like, *Should I have mentioned that I wrote that first book in less than a month? Will the reader think I am conceited or that the book was bad?*). On this project, the hours burrowed away at my home office, on a plane, in an airport, or in a producer's car piled up. The reporting trips, the writing time, all the ruminating and endless cud-chewing was particularly taxing on my family.

On the other end of this cud-chewing was my editor, Yaniv Soha of Doubleday. The manuscript for this book was completed within a week of his wife, Jess, giving birth to their angelic Ayla. Poor guy, his first task after returning from paternity leave was tackling this edit. A good editor is like a careful gardener, who sprinkles nutrients through long conversations, then, once words sprout on the page, nurtures certain passages and prunes back tangents that won't survive. In that department Yaniv has a green thumb, but he is also exquisitely sensitive and monumentally dedicated, and for both those traits I am especially indebted.

If Yaniv is the tender gardener, my agent Byrd Leavell of UTA helped sow the seed. He was enthusiastic about this project from the moment he heard me describe my panics. I initially offered Leavell a messy idea, which he helped me mold into something that would eventually become the backbone of this book—with the full support of his boss and head of UTA, Jay Sures, who was one of the first people in whom I confided about my panics and who was a tireless supporter of this project. Hannah Kekst helped me with one of the tasks I dreaded most, the organization of this book's bibliography and the many footnotes and endnotes.

So much is owed to the dozens of people who generously gave of their time. From strangers who lent an ear on a plane to all the good people in those panic attack support groups. Randy Nesse was kind and generous and remarkably patient with my shifting schedule. His book *Good Reasons for Bad Feelings* was seminal in my depathologizing of panic. I learned about Nesse by mining the knowledge of people like evolutionary psychologists Glenn Geher and Daniel Glass. Nesse and Robert Sapolsky kindly weighed in on drafts of this book, helping me with the science.

Sapolsky also submitted to multiple conversations and took time out from writing his own book to teach me what must have seemed pathetically rudimentary to him—the ABCs of anxiety in apes and humans (and dinosaurs). Mike Telch welcomed me to his home and the world of CBT—and let me breathe all the CO_2 I could ever want (and more). We continue to speak, and he remains a dear friend. Mitch Prinstein not only contributed to this book in multiple interviews but served as a sounding board and voice of reason. Same with Ellen Vora, who took time out from vacations and conferences to talk, and dispensed her wisdom in near-flawless sound bites.

I am indebted to the folks on my Peruvian ayahuasca retreat, who knew I was writing a book and yet generously introduced me to their sequined harlequin gremlins, their serpent witches, and their gods.

I spent many hours talking with friends Michael Solomon and Lane Jaffe about what path this story should take, how it should be told, and, with Michael especially, what it should be called. Years ago, Dan Harris was one of the first people I ever told about my panics, and he was one of the last people I interviewed for this book. I am indebted to his kindness to me while at ABC and his insight since then.

At ABC, my managers David Herndon and Bonnie McLean supported me in every way they could. The ABC brass, led by company president Kim Godwin and Tanya Menton, championed the project and read early drafts, providing key feedback. So did the many producers and other colleagues, like Sony Salzman and Dr. Nick Nissen, who offered scientific feedback and advice.

My wife, Daphna, uncomplainingly bore the brunt of it. From the humiliation of my suspension to the grind of many edits. There were many weekends in which I traveled to report or to journey psychedelically. Sometimes it was a lot. Throughout, Daphna offered perspective, urging me to bring more of the personal and to venture deeper—tapping places it was not always comfortable for me to go (publicly). Daphi, I am forever indebted.

The kids frequently asked the completely reasonable question "When are you going to be done with this book?" but never "*Why* are you doing this book anyway?" With his sister Libby's help, my son Ben even offered a few samples of cover art, hoping to get the ball rolling. As most parents will attest, it is your kids who make you want to become a better, healthier human and a more whole one.

Notes

The majority of this book is drawn from interviews I conducted between the years 2020 and 2022. I have tried whenever possible to credit my interviewees in the text as well as below. Please note that due to the controversial nature of some of the practices I've described in this book and the sensitive personal information that my interview subjects often divulged, I have, in several instances, changed a subject's name or their identifying features.

PROLOGUE

6   More than a quarter of all Americans: Kessler et al., "The Epidemiology of Panic Attacks, Panic Disorder, and Agoraphobia."

6   Some panic experts believe: Telch interview, April 1, 2021.

7   Panic attacks so convincingly: Musey et al., "Anxiety About Anxiety."

7   over 2.5 million Americans: Centers for Disease Control and Prevention, "National Hospital Ambulatory Medical Care Survey: 2018 Emergency Department Summary Tables."

8   Diagnoses, both psychological and physiological: Ackerman, "From Chemistry to Circuitry."

8   At the time of this writing: Scheffer et al., "A Connectome and Analysis of the Adult *Drosophila* Central Brain"; Herculano-Houzel, "The Remarkable, Yet Not Extraordinary, Human Brain."

8   clarity of a diagnosis: Kessler, Berglund, and Demler, "Lifetime Prevalence and Age-of-Onset Distributions of *DSM-IV* Disorders."

8   The human brain is a marvel: Kováč, "The 20 W Sleep-Walkers."

CHAPTER 1: TEXTBOOK PANIC

18   Fear helps us survive: Judson Brewer interviewed by Matt Gutman, February 9, 2023.

19   anxiety about having panic: Kessler et al., "The Epidemiology of Panic Attacks, Panic Disorder, and Agoraphobia."

19   It is so pervasive that: Muda, "Relationship Between Glossophobia and Emotional Intelligence."

19   The National Institute of Mental Health: National Institute of Mental Health, "Social Anxiety Disorder."

21   Even then, doctors found nothing: Centers for Disease Control and Prevention, "Heart Disease Facts"; Musey et al., "Anxiety About Anxiety."

21   That could mean more than 2.6 million: Centers for Disease Control and Prevention, "National Hospital Ambulatory Medical Care Survey: 2019 Emergency Department Summary Tables."

21   One study sponsored by: Karaca and Moore, "Costs of Emergency Department Visits for Mental and Substance Use Disorders."

22   clinically defined as exposure to: Pai, Suris, and North, "Posttraumatic Stress Disorder in the *DSM-5*."

22   you are far more likely to have: Kessler et al., "The Epidemiology of Panic Attacks, Panic Disorder, and Agoraphobia."

22   Surveys consistently find: Kessler et al., "The Epidemiology of Panic Attacks, Panic Disorder, and Agoraphobia."

22   Either way, regardless of gender: Centers for Disease Control and Prevention, "Excessive Alcohol Use and Men's Health."

22   According to that Indiana University study: Musey et al., "Anxiety About Anxiety."

22   a patient's body, not mind: Musey et al., "Anxiety About Anxiety."

23   untold numbers of patients: Kessler et al., "The Epidemiology of Panic Attacks, Panic Disorder, and Agoraphobia."

27   Some psychologists and neurologists: Nesse interview, September 30, 2021.

27   That's when the brain's command center: Sapolsky interview, September 7, 2022.

28   In freezing, the heart rate: Roelofs, "Freeze for Action."

28   This is called an extreme: Bracha, Bienvenu, and Eaton, "Testing the Paleolithic-Human-Warfare Hypothesis."

29   an ability to convincingly play dead: Bracha, "Freeze, Flight, Fight, Fright, Faint."

29   I began to sweat: Telch interview, May 2021.

31   The etymology of the word *panic*: Merriam-Webster, "The Mythological Origin of 'Panic.'"

31   "to prevent panic, hysteria": Fairchild, Johns, and Sivaramakrishnan, "A Brief History of Panic."

31   They were, it was said: Tasca, Rapetti, Carta, and Fadda, "Women and Hysteria in the History of Mental Health."

32   To balance those "humors": Fotiou and Gearin, "Purging and the Body in the Therapeutic Use of Ayahuasca."

34   a stunning achievement: Hulse et al., "A connectome of the *Drosophila* central complex."

34   An article published in 2019: Tompa, "5 Unsolved Mysteries About the Brain."

34   If we can't even figure out: Sapolsky interview, September 7, 2022.

34   "With drugs like opioids": Tompa, "5 Unsolved Mysteries About the Brain."

34   For many folks with depression: Cipriani et al., "Comparative Efficacy and Acceptability of 21 Antidepressant Drugs."

35   A recent survey by the World Health Organization: World Health Organization, "Depression and Other Common Mental Health Disorders," 10–14.

35   It could well be that rates: Hofmann and Hinton, "Cross-Cultural Aspects of Anxiety Disorders."

35   But it's also possible: Musey et al., "Anxiety About Anxiety."

CHAPTER 2: KEEPING THE SECRET

45   who are incapable of accepting: Bravata et al., "Prevalence, Predictors, and Treatment of Impostor Syndrome."

CHAPTER 3: THE GOOD PANIC

66   A sauropod couldn't be anxious: Sapolsky interview, March 9, 2021.

67   Chemically, early apes: Sapolsky interview, September 7, 2022.

67   That's better than expending hundreds: Cole, "Assessing the Calorific Significance of Episodes in Human Cannibalism."

70   Those baboon bosses find: Gesquiere et al., "Life at the Top."

72   Scientists believe that runaway: Nesse interview, September 27, 2021; Sapolsky interview, March 9, 2021.

CHAPTER 4: A THOUSAND FALSE ALARMS

75   Given the reportedly surging anxiety: Curtin, "State Suicide Rates Among Adolescents and Young Adults," 1–6.

75   Hence the appeal: Towle, "Human Ancestors Had the Same Dental Problems as Us."

76   The fossil record: Burger, Baudisch, and Vaupel, "Human Mortality Improvement in Evolutionary Context."

76   That's to say nothing: Spikins, "The Stone Age Origins of Autism."

76   believe, multiple studies: Kranioti, Grigorescu, and Harvati, "State of the Art Forensic Techniques"; Roser, "Ethnographic and Archaeological Evidence on Violent Deaths."

76   This includes starvation, falling rocks: Sapolsky interview, March 9, 2021.

77   Evolutionary psychologists believe: Christakis interview, October 20, 2021.

77   This is why, before the invention: Sterelny, "Language, Gesture, Skill."

77   The fine-tuning of fear: Christakis interview, October 20, 2021.

78   In fact, grandmothers: Lee, "Rethinking the Evolutionary Theory of Aging"; O'Connell, Hawkes, and Blurton Jones, "Grandmothering and the Evolution of *Homo erectus*."

79   Being able to harmoniously: Lieberman interview, September 12, 2021.

79   Over time our bodies: Lieberman interview, September 12, 2021.

79   Welcome to the world: Sterelny, "Cooperation, Culture, and Conflict," 46.

79   But be a serial shirker: Lohse and Waichman, "The Effects of Contemporaneous Peer Punishment on Cooperation."

80   *Listen, Zek, you saw that*: Rand, Arbesman, and Christakis, "Dynamic Social Networks Promote Cooperation in Experiments with Humans."

80   Furthermore, studies have shown: Wesselmann, Nairne, and Williams, "An Evolutionary Social Psychological Approach to Studying the Effects of Ostracism."

80   Like it or not, tens of thousands: Gilbert, "Evolution and Social Anxiety."

81   so central to our human survival: Eisenberger, Jarcho, Lieberman, and Naliboff, "An Experimental Study of Shared Sensitivity."

81   The bigger the social rejection: Eisenberger, Lieberman, and Williams, "Does Rejection Hurt?"

82   it's not just expulsion or rejection: Sapolsky interview, March 13,
            2021; Christakis interview, October 20, 2021.
84   "sudden foolish frights": From Plutarch's *The Philosophie*: "Sud-
            den foolish frights, without any certeine cause, which they call
            Panique Terrores."

CHAPTER 5: DISCLOSURE
96   Even if you count only: National Institute of Mental Health,
            "Panic Disorder."
96   there are over 123,000 AA groups: Alcoholics Anonymous, "A.A.
            Around the World"; Timko et al., "Al-Anon Family Groups."
100   If we drove as well: Centers for Disease Control and Prevention,
            "Motor Vehicle Crash Deaths."

CHAPTER 6: WHEN THE DOCTOR SEES YOU
108   Chronic anxiety can increase: Lewis, "Psychological Distress and
            Death from Cardiovascular Disease."
109   It ruins quality of sleep: DeWall and Bushman, "Social Acceptance
            and Rejection."
109   It's little wonder that a meta-survey: Kowalski et al., "K-12,
            College/University, and Mass Shootings."
114   In some cases, they evidently trigger: Callaway and Grob, "Aya-
            huasca Preparations and Serotonin Reuptake Inhibitors."
115   "Our comprehensive review": Moncrieff et al., "The Serotonin
            Theory of Depression."
115   depression "may discourage": Moncrieff et al., "The Serotonin The-
            ory of Depression."
116   They can be much more addictive: Moncrieff et al., "The Sero-
            tonin Theory of Depression."

CHAPTER 7: LOBSTER CLAWS AND MUSHROOMS
127   One such study: Mitchell et al., "MDMA-Assisted Therapy for
            Severe PTSD."

CHAPTER 8: THE DOSE MAKES THE POISON
138   "That's followed by . . . a dream state": "Dreams, visions and
            diarrhea: What to expect if you take ayahuasca," CBC Radio,
            April 24, 2018.
138   After hearing that I'd been prescribed Paxil: Callaway and Grob,
            "Ayahuasca Preparations and Serotonin Reuptake Inhibitors."

Bibliography

Ackerman, Sandra. "From Chemistry to Circuitry." In *Discovering the Brain*, ed. Sandra Ackerman for the Institute of Medicine, National Academy of Sciences, 67–85. Washington, D.C.: National Academies Press, 1992.

Ait-Daoud, Nassima, Allan Scott Hamby, Sana Sharma, and Derek Blevins. "A Review of Alprazolam Use, Misuse, and Withdrawal." *Journal of Addictive Medicine* 12, no. 1 (February 2018): 4–10. https://doi.org/10.1097/ADM.0000000000000350.

Alcoholics Anonymous. "A.A. Around the World." www.aa.org.

American Psychological Association. "What Is Cognitive Behavioral Therapy?" www.apa.org.

Benagiano, Giuseppe, and Maurizio Mori. "The Origins of Human Sexuality: Procreation or Recreation?" *Reproductive BioMedicine Online* 18, suppl. 1 (2009): 50–59. https://doi.org/10.1016/s1472-6483(10)60116-2.

Bracha, H. Stefan. "Freeze, Flight, Fight, Fright, Faint: Adaptationist Perspectives on the Acute Stress Response Spectrum." *CNS Spectrums* 9, no. 9 (September 2004): 679–85. https://doi.org/10.1017/s1092852900001954.

Bracha, H. Stefan, O. Joseph Bienvenu, and William W. Eaton. "Testing the Paleolithic-Human-Warfare Hypothesis of Blood-Injection Phobia in the Baltimore ECA Follow-Up Study—Towards a More Etiologically-Based Conceptualization for *DSM-V*." *Journal of Affective Disorders* 97, no. 1–3 (January 2007): 1–4. https://doi.org/10.1016/j.jad.2006.06.014.

Bravata, Dena M., Sharon A. Watts, Autumn L. Keefer, Divya K. Madhusudhan, Katie T. Taylor, Dani M. Clark, Ross S. Nelson, et al. "Prevalence, Predictors, and Treatment of Impostor Syndrome: A Systematic Review." *Journal of General Internal Medicine* 35, no. 4 (April 2020): 1252–75. https://doi.org/10.1007/s11606-019-05364-1.

Brewer, Judson. *Unwinding Anxiety: New Science Shows How to Break the Cycles of Worry and Fear to Heal Your Mind*. New York, NY: Avery, 2021.

Burger, Oskar, Annette Baudisch, and James W. Vaupel. "Human Mortality Improvement in Evolutionary Context." *Proceedings of the National Academy of Sciences* 109, no. 44 (October 2012): 18210–14. https://doi .org/10.1073/pnas.1215627109.

Bylsma, Lauren M., Asmir Gračanin, and Ad J.J.M. Vingerhoets. "The Neurobiology of Human Crying." *Clinical Autonomic Research* 29, no. 1 (February 2019): 63–73. https://doi.org/10.1007/s10286-018-0526-y.

Callaway, James C., and Charles S. Grob. "Ayahuasca Preparations and Serotonin Reuptake Inhibitors: A Potential Combination for Severe Adverse Interactions." *Journal of Psychoactive Drugs* 30, no. 4 (October 1998): 367–69. https://doi.org/10.1080/02791072.1998.10399712.

Carrier, Scott. *Running After Antelope*. Berkeley: Counterpoint, 2002.

Centers for Disease Control and Prevention. "Excessive Alcohol Use and Men's Health." www.cdc.gov/alcohol.

Centers for Disease Control and Prevention. "Heart Disease Facts." www .cdc.gov.

Centers for Disease Control and Prevention. "Motor Vehicle Crash Deaths: How Is the US Doing?" www.cdc.gov.

Centers for Disease Control and Prevention. "National Hospital Ambulatory Medical Care Survey: Emergency Department Fact Sheet." www .cdc.gov.

Centers for Disease Control and Prevention. "National Hospital Ambulatory Medical Care Survey: 2018 Emergency Department Summary Tables." www.cdc.gov.

Centers for Disease Control and Prevention. "National Hospital Ambulatory Medical Care Survey: 2019 Emergency Department Summary Tables." www.cdc.gov.

Centers for Disease Control and Prevention. "Road Traffic Injuries and Deaths—A Global Problem." www.cdc.gov.

Chapais, Bernard. *Primeval Kinship: How Pair-Bonding Gave Birth to Human Society*. Cambridge: Harvard University Press, 2008.

Christakis, Nicholas. Interviewed by Matt Gutman, October 20, 2021.

Cipriani, Andrea, Toshi A. Furukawa, Georgia Salanti, Anna Chaimani, Lauren Z. Atkinson, Yusuke Ogawa, Stefan Leucht, et al. "Comparative Efficacy and Acceptability of 21 Antidepressant Drugs for the Acute Treatment of Adults with Major Depressive Disorder: A Systematic Review and Network Meta-Analysis." *The Lancet* 391, no. 10128 (February 2018): 1357–66. https://doi.org/10.1016/S0140-6736(17)32802-7.

Cole, James. "Assessing the Calorific Significance of Episodes in Human Cannibalism in the Paleolithic." *Scientific Reports* 7 (2017): 44707. https://doi.org/10.1038/srep44707.

Coste, Joël, and Bernard Granger. "Mental Disorders in Ancient Medical Writings: Methods of Characterization and Application to French Consultations (16th–18th Centuries)." *Annales médico-psychologiques, revue psychiatrique* 172, no. 8 (October 2014): 625–33. https://doi.org/10.1016/j.amp.2013.07.006.

Crocq, Marc-Antoine. "A History of Anxiety: From Hippocrates to *DSM*." *Dialogues in Clinical Neuroscience* 17, no. 3 (September 2015): 319–25. https://doi.org/10.31887/DCNS.2015.17.3/macrocq.

Curtin, Sally C. "State Suicide Rates Among Adolescents and Young Adults Aged 10–24: United States, 2000–2018." *National Vital Statistics Reports* 69, no. 11 (September 2020). www.cdc.gov.

D'Acquisto, Fulvio, and Alice Hamilton. "Cardiovascular and Immunological Implications of Social Distancing in the Context of COVID-19." *Cardiovascular Research* 116, no. 10 (August 2021): e129–e131. https://doi.org/10.1093/cvr/cvaa167.

Davidson, Richard J., and Antoine Lutz. "Buddha's Brain: Neuroplasticity and Meditation." *IEEE Signal Processing Magazine* 25, no. 1 (January 2008): 174–76. https://doi.org/10.1109/msp.2008.4431873.

DeWall, C. Nathan, and Brad J. Bushman. "Social Acceptance and Rejection: The Sweet and the Bitter." *Current Directions in Psychological Science* 20, no. 4 (2011): 256–60. https://doi.org/10.1177/0963721411417545.

Eisenberger, Naomi I., Johanna M. Jarcho, Matthew D. Lieberman, and Bruce D. Naliboff. "An Experimental Study of Shared Sensitivity to Physical Pain and Social Rejection." *Pain* 126, no. 1 (December 2006): 132–38. https://doi.org/10.1016/j.pain.2006.06.024.

Eisenberger, Naomi I., Matthew D. Lieberman, and Kipling D. Williams. "Does Rejection Hurt? An fMRI Study of Exclusion." *Science* 302, no. 5643 (October 2003): 290–92. http://doi.org/10.1126/science.1089134.

Ermakova, Anna O., Fiona Dunbar, James Rucker, and Matthew W. Johnson. "A Narrative Synthesis of Research with 5-MeO-DMT." *Journal of Psychopharmacology* 36, no. 3 (October 2021): 273–94. https://doi.org/10.1177/02698811211050543.

Fairchild, Amy L., David Merritt Johns, and Kavita Sivaramakrishnan. "A Brief History of Panic." *New York Times,* January 28, 2013.

Fessler, Daniel M. T., Leonid B. Tiokhin, Colin Holbrook, Matthew M. Gervais, and Jeffrey K. Snyder. "Foundations of the Crazy Bastard Hypothesis: Nonviolent Physical Risk-Taking Enhances Conceptualized Formidability." *Evolution and Human Behavior* 35, no. 1 (January 2014): 26–33. https://doi.org/10.1016/j.evolhumbehav.2013.09.003.

Fotiou, Evgenia, and Alex K. Gearin. "Purging and the Body in the Therapeutic Use of Ayahuasca." *Social Science and Medicine* 239 (August 2019): 112532. https://doi.org/10.1016/j.socscimed.2019.112532.

Francuski, Xavier. "Why We Strive for Ego Death with Psychedelics." Kahpi: The Ayahuasca Hub, November 5, 2018. https://kahpi.net.

Gallup, Gordon G., Jr., Richard F. Nash, Nelson H. Donegan, and Michael K. McClure. "The Immobility Response: A Predator-Induced Reaction in Chickens." *Psychological Record* 21 (1971): 513–19. https://doi.org/10.1007/BF03394049.

Gavrilets, Sergey. "Human Origins and the Transition from Promiscuity to Pair-Bonding." *Proceedings of the National Academy of Sciences* 109, no. 25 (May 2012): 9923–28. https://doi.org/10.1073/pnas.1200717109.

Gesquiere, Laurence R., Niki H. Learn, M. Carolina M. Simao, Patrick O. Onyango, Susan C. Alberts, and Jeanne Altmann. "Life at the Top: Rank and Stress in Wild Male Baboons." *Science* 333, no. 6040 (July 2011): 357–60. https://doi.org/10.1126/science.1207120.

Gilbert, Paul. "Evolution and Social Anxiety: The Role of Attraction, Social Competition, and Social Hierarchies." *Psychiatric Clinics of North America* 24, no. 4 (December 2001): 723–51. https://doi.org/10.1016/s0193-953x(05)70260-4.

Herculano-Houzel, Suzana. "The Remarkable, Yet Not Extraordinary, Human Brain as a Scaled-Up Primate Brain and Its Associated Cost." *Proceedings of the National Academy of Sciences* 109, suppl. 1 (June 2012): 10661–68. https://doi.org/10.1073/pnas.1201895109.

Hofmann, Stefan G., and Devon E. Hinton. "Cross-Cultural Aspects of Anxiety Disorders." *Current Psychiatry Reports* 16, no. 6 (June 2014): 450. https://doi.org/10.1007/s11920-014-0450-3.

Hulse, Brad K., Hannah Haberkern, Romain Franconville, Daniel Turner-Evans, Shin-ya Takemura, Tanya Wolff, Marcella Noorman, et al. "A connectome of the *Drosophila* central complex reveals network motifs suitable for flexible navigation and context-dependent action selection." *eLife* 10 (October 2021): e66039. https://elifesciences.org/articles/66039.

Karaca, Zeynal, and Brian J. Moore. "Costs of Emergency Department Visits for Mental and Substance Use Disorders in the United States, 2017." Statistical Brief #257, 2020. Healthcare Cost and Utilization Project, Agency for Healthcare Research and Quality. www.hcup-us.ahrq.gov.

Kessler, Ronald C., Patricia Berglund, and Olga Demler. "Lifetime Prevalence and Age-of-Onset Distributions of *DSM-IV* Disorders in the National Comorbidity Survey Replication." *Archives of General Psychiatry* 62, no. 6 (June 2005): 593–602. https://doi.org/10.1001/archpsyc.62.6.593.

Kessler, Ronald C., Wai Tat Chiu, Robert Jin, Ayelet Meron Ruscio, Katherine Shear, and Ellen E. Walters. "The Epidemiology of Panic Attacks, Panic Disorder, and Agoraphobia in the National Comorbidity Survey Replication." *Archives of General Psychiatry* 63, no. 4 (April 2006): 415–24. https://doi.org/10.1001/archpsyc.63.4.415.

Kováč, Ladislav. "The 20 W Sleep-Walkers." *EMBO Reports* 11, no. 1 (January 2010): 2. https://doi.org/10.1038/embor.2009.266.

Kowalski, Robin Marie, Mark Leary, Tyler Hendley, Kaitlyn Rubley, Catherine Chapman, Hannah Chitty, Hailey Carroll, et al. "K-12, College/University, and Mass Shootings: Similarities and Differences." *Journal of Social Psychology* 161, no. 6 (November 2021): 753–78. https://doi.org/10.1080/00224545.2021.1900047.

Kramer, Karen L., and Andrew F. Russell. "Was Monogamy a Key Step on the Hominin Road? Reevaluating the Monogamy Hypothesis in the Evolution of Cooperative Breeding." *Evolutionary Anthropology* 24, no. 2 (March 2015): 73–83. https://doi.org/10.1002/evan.21445.

Kranioti, Elena, Dan Grigorescu, and Katerina Harvati. "State of the Art Forensic Techniques Reveal Evidence of Interpersonal Violence ca. 30,000 Years Ago." *PLoS ONE* 14, no. 7 (July 2019): e0216718. https://doi.org/10.1371/journal.pone.0216718.

Kross, Ethan. *Chatter: The Voice in Our Head, Why It Matters, and How to Harness It*. New York, NY: Crown, 2021.

Lee, Ronald D. "Rethinking the Evolutionary Theory of Aging: Transfers, Not Births, Shape Senescence in Social Species." *Proceedings of the National Academy of Sciences* 100, no. 16 (August 2003): 9637–42. https://doi.org/10.1073/pnas.1530303100.

LePera, Nicole. *How to Do the Work: Recognize Your Patterns, Heal from Your Past, and Create Your Self*. New York, NY: Harper Wave, 2021.

Lewis, Glyn. "Psychological Distress and Death from Cardiovascular Disease." *BMJ* 345 (July 2012): e5177. https://doi.org/10.1136/bmj.e5177.

Lieberman, Dan. Interviewed by Matt Gutman, September 12, 2021.

Lohse, Johannes, and Israel Waichman. "The Effects of Contemporaneous Peer Punishment on Cooperation with the Future." *Nature Communications* 11 (2020): 1815. https://doi.org/10.1038/s41467-020-15661-7.

Maté, Daniel, and Gabor Maté. *The Myth of Normal: Trauma, Illness, and Healing in a Toxic Culture*. New York, NY: Avery, 2022.

Merriam-Webster. "The Mythological Origin of 'Panic.'" Word History blog. www.merriam-webster.com.

Mitchell, Jennifer M., Michael Bogenschutz, Alia Lilienstein, Charlotte Harrison, Sarah Kleiman, Kelly Parker-Guilbert, Marcela Ot'alora G., et al. "MDMA-Assisted Therapy for Severe PTSD: A Randomized, Double-Blind, Placebo-Controlled Phase 3 Study." *Nature Medicine* 27 (June 2021): 1025–33. https://doi.org/10.1038/s41591-021-01336-3.

Moncrieff, Joanna, Ruth E. Cooper, Tom Stockmann, Simone Amendola, Michael P. Hengartner, and Mark A. Horowitz. "The Serotonin Theory of Depression: A Systematic Umbrella Review of the Evidence." *Molecular Psychology* (2022). https://doi.org/10.1038/s41380-022-01661-0.

Muda, Tengku Elmi Azlina Tengku. "Relationship Between Glossophobia and Emotional Intelligence Among Asasi Pintar Students." *Journal of Social Sciences Research* 6 (2018): 223–29. https://doi.org/10.32861/jssr.spi6.223.229.

Murrough, James W., Dan V. Iosifescu, Lee C. Chang, Rayan K. Al Jurdi, Charles M. Green, Andrew M. Perez, Syed Iqbal, et al. "Antidepressant Efficacy of Ketamine in Treatment-Resistant Major Depression: A Two-Site Randomized Controlled Trial." *American Journal of Psychiatry* 170, no. 10 (October 2013): 1134–42. https://doi.org/10.1176/appi.ajp.2013.13030392.

Musey, Paul I., Jr., John A. Lee, Cassandra A. Hall, and Jeffrey A. Kline. "Anxiety About Anxiety: A Survey of Emergency Department Provider Beliefs and Practices Regarding Anxiety-Associated Low Risk Chest Pain." *BMC Emergency Medicine* 18 (March 2018): 10. https://doi.org/10.1186/s12873-018-0161-x.

National Institute of Mental Health. "Panic Disorder." www.nimh.nih.gov/health/statistics/panic-disorder.

National Institute of Mental Health. "Social Anxiety Disorder." www.nimh.nih.gov/health/statistics/social-anxiety-disorder.

Nesse, Randy. Interviewed by Matt Gutman, September 27, 2021.

O'Connell, J. F., K. Hawkes, and N. G. Blurton Jones. "Grandmothering and the Evolution of *Homo erectus.*" *Journal of Human Evolution* 36, no. 5 (May 1999): 461–85. https://doi.org/10.1006/jhev.1998.0285.

Pai, Anushka, Alina M. Suris, and Carol S. North. "Posttraumatic Stress Disorder in the *DSM-5:* Controversy, Change, and Conceptual Considerations." *Behavioral Sciences* 7, no. 1 (March 2017): 7. https://doi.org/10.3390/bs7010007.

Plutarch. *The Philosophie, commonlie called, The Morals.* Translated by Philemon Holland. London: Arnold Hatfield, 1603.

Prinstein, Mitch. Interviewed by Matt Gutman, April 2, 2021.

Rand, David G., Samuel Arbesman, and Nicholas A. Christakis. "Dynamic Social Networks Promote Cooperation in Experiments with Humans." *Proceedings of the National Academy of Sciences* 108, no. 48 (November 2011): 19193–98. https://doi.org/10.1073/pnas.1108243108.

Roelofs, Karen. "Freeze for Action: Neurobiological Mechanisms in Animal and Human Freezing." *Philosophical Transactions of the Royal Society B* 372, no. 1718 (April 2017): 20160206. https://doi.org/10.1098/rstb.2016.0206.

Ronson, Jon. *So You've Been Publicly Shamed.* New York, NY: Riverhead Books, 2015.

Roser, Max. "Ethnographic and Archaeological Evidence on Violent Deaths." *Our World in Data,* August 2, 2013. https://ourworldindata.org/.

Santomauro, Damian F., Ana M. Mantilla Herrera, Jamileh Shadid, Peng Zheng, Charlie Ashbaugh, David M. Pigott, et al. "Global Prevalence and Burden of Depressive and Anxiety Disorders in 204 Countries and Territories in 2020 due to the COVID-19 Pandemic." *The Lancet* 398, no. 101312 (November 2021): 1700–1712. https://doi.org/10.1016/S0140-6736(21)02143-7.

Sapolsky, Robert. Interviewed by Matt Gutman, March 9, 2021; March 13, 2021; September 7, 2022.

Sapolsky, Robert M. *Behave: The Biology of Humans at Our Best and Worst.* New York, NY: Penguin Press, 2017.

Sapolsky, Robert M. *A Primate's Memoir.* New York, NY: Scribner, 2001.

Sapolsky, Robert M. *Why Zebras Don't Get Ulcers.* Third Edition. New York, NY: Holt Paperbacks, 2004.

Scheffer, Louis K., C. Chan Xu, Michal Januszewski, Zhiyuan Lu, Shinya Takemura, Kenneth J. Hayworth, Gary B. Huang, et al. "A Connectome and Analysis of the Adult *Drosophila* Central Brain." *eLife* 9 (September 2020): e57443. https://doi.org/10.7554/eLife.57443.

Spikins, Penny. "The Stone Age Origins of Autism." In *Recent Advances in Autism Spectrum Disorders*, ed. Michael Fitzgerald, 3–24. London: IntechOpen, 2013.

Sterelny, Kim. "Cooperation, Culture, and Conflict." *British Journal for the Philosophy of Science* 67, no. 1 (March 2016): 31–58. https://doi.org/10.1093/bjps/axu024.

Sterelny, Kim. "Language, Gesture, Skill: The Co-Evolutionary Foundations of Language." *Philosophical Transactions of the Royal Society B* 367, no. 1599 (August 2012): 2141–51. https://doi.org/10.1098/rstb.2012.0116.

Tasca, Cecilia, Mariangela Rapetti, Mauro Giovanni Carta, and Bianca Fadda. "Women and Hysteria in the History of Mental Health." *Clinical Practice and Epidemiology in Mental Health* 8 (October 2012): 110–19. https://doi.org/10.2174/1745017901208010110.

Telch, Michael. Interviewed by Matt Gutman, April 1, 2021; May 2021.

Timko, Christine, Ruth Cronkite, Lee Ann Kaskutas, Alexandre Laudet, Jeffrey Roth, and Rudolf H. Moos. "Al-Anon Family Groups: Newcomers and Members." *Journal of Studies on Alcohol and Drugs* 74, no. 6 (November 2013): 965–76. https://doi.org/10.15288/jsad.2013.74.965.

Tompa, Rachel. "5 Unsolved Mysteries About the Brain." Allen Institute, March 14, 2019. https://alleninstitute.org.

Towle, Ian. "Human Ancestors Had the Same Dental Problems as Us—Even Without Fizzy Drinks and Sweets." *The Conversation*, March 1, 2018. https://theconversation.com/.

Wesselmann, Eric D., James S. Nairne, and Kipling D. Williams. "An Evolutionary Social Psychological Approach to Studying the Effects of Ostracism." *Journal of Social, Evolutionary, and Cultural Psychology* 6, no. 3 (2012): 309–28. https://doi.org/10.1037/h0099249.

World Health Organization. "Depression and Other Common Mental Health Disorders." 2017. https://apps.who.int.